Migration and Health

Studies of the Biosocial Society

General Editor: **Catherine Panter-Brick,** Professor of Anthropology, Yale University

The Biosocial Society is an international academic society engaged in fostering understanding of human biological and social diversity. It draws its membership from a wide range of academic disciplines, particularly those engaged in "boundary disciplines" at the intersection between the natural and social sciences, such as bio-cultural anthropology, medical sociology, demography, social medicine, the history of science and bioethics. The aim of this series is to promote interdisciplinary research on how biology and society interact to shape human experience and to serve as advanced texts for undergraduate and postgraduate students.

Volume 10
Migration and Health: Challenging the Borders of Belonging, Care, and Policy
Edited by Nadia El-Shaarawi and Stéphanie Larchanché

Volume 9
Understanding Conflicts about Wildlife: A Biosocial Approach
Edited by Catherine M. Hill, Amanda D. Webber and Nancy E.C. Priston

Volume 8
Health and Difference: Rendering Human Engagement in Colonial Engagements
Edited by Alexandra Widmer and Veronika Lipphardt

Volume 7
Ethics in the Field: Contemporary Challenges
Edited by Jeremy MacClancy and Agustín Fuentes

Volume 6
Identity Politics after DNA: Re/Creating Categories of Difference and Belonging
Edited by Katharina Schramm, David Skinner, and Richard Rottenburg

Volume 5
Human Diet and Nutrition in Biocultural Perspective: Past Meets Present
Edited by Tina Moffat and Tracy Prowse

Volume 4
Centralizing Fieldwork: Critical Perspectives from Primatology, Biological and Social Anthropology
Edited by Jeremy MacClancy and Agustín Fuentes

Volume 3
Substitute Parents:Biological and Social Perspective on Alloparenting in Human Societies
Edited by Gillian Bentley and Ruth Mace

Volume 2
Health, Risk, and Adversity
Edited by Catherine Panter-Brick and Agustín Fuentes

Volume 1
Race, Ethnicity, and Nation: Perspectives from Kinship and Genetics
Edited by Peter Wade

Migration and Health

Challenging the Borders of Belonging, Care, and Policy

Edited by
Nadia El-Shaarawi and Stéphanie Larchanché

berghahn
NEW YORK • OXFORD
www.berghahnbooks.com

First published in 2022 by
Berghahn Books
www.berghahnbooks.com

Library of Congress Cataloging-in-Publication Data

Names: El-Shaarawi, Nadia, editor. | Larchanché, Stéphanie, editor.
Title: Migration and health : challenging the borders of belonging, care, and policy / edited by Nadia El-Shaarawi and Stéphanie Larchanché.
Description: New York : Berghahn Books, [2022] | Series: Studies of the biosocial society ; volume 10 | Includes bibliographical references and index.
Identifiers: LCCN 2022012989 (print) | LCCN 2022012990 (ebook) | ISBN 9781800735019 (hardback) | ISBN 9781800735026 (ebook)
Subjects: LCSH: Immigrants--Medical care. | Emigration and immigration—Health aspects.
Classification: LCC RA408.M5 M53 2022 (print) | LCC RA408.M5 (ebook) | DDC 362.1086/912—dc23/eng/20220330
LC record available at https://lccn.loc.gov/2022012989
LC ebook record available at https://lccn.loc.gov/2022012990

British Library Cataloguing in Publication Data

A catalogue record for this book is available from the British Library

ISBN 978-1-80073-501-9 hardback
ISBN 978-1-80073-502-6 ebook

https://doi.org/10.3167/9781800735019

Contents

Foreword

Catherine Panter-Brick

Take a journey through this book, a journey through time and place, a journey to identify the borders of belonging and discern the frontiers of knowledge on migration and health. As I write this foreword, we have just marked the one-year anniversary of the COVID-19 pandemic. So many times over this past year have we confronted COVID-19-related lockdowns, loss and hardships, risks to health and well-being, and inequities born of social and economic policy—but also grassroots solidarity and caregiving. I cannot think of a better time to reflect upon issues of migration, health, belonging, care, and policy, especially from an ethnographic lens. Of course, scholarship on migration and health predates all concerns with the COVID-19 pandemic; yet the latter has starkly reminded us that global migration brings a whole host of challenges to people and policy. It has also reminded us that health vulnerabilities are never asocial and responses to health care are never apolitical; and so we need to knit together the biological, the social, and the political, as this volume does. Indeed, because we often have disciplinary blind spots when it comes to health, health care, and migrants, we need to challenge the borders of knowledge, practice, and action to bring about fresh conversations about migration and health.

A journey through this book might prompt reflection on epistemic borders. We might better understand "borders" in terms of social inclusion, contested exclusion, and relational care, rather than in terms of the geographies of health. We might think anew of borders as systems of beliefs and practices, presenting real challenges to health and struggles in the pursuit of healthcare, rather than just places to be crossed, mapped, and cataloged; for example, we might ask which kinds of immigration policies are contested, which kinds of borders are policed or defended, which kinds of people are excluded from care, and why or when are they consequential for health care equity. Borders are often intended to serve the logic of social difference and colonial hierarchy, but they also engender new social imaginaries and new encounters and ideas about ways to connect with each other, care for each other, transform our world, and broaden our lived experiences.

This book is situated within the Berghahn series that promotes interdisciplinary research on how biology and society interact to structure human experience. The aim is to offer biosocial and biocultural texts that engage boundary disciplines across the natural sciences, social sciences, and humanities, to serve as research and teaching texts on issues of specific importance. I am very proud that scholars from a wide range of institutions, sub-disciplines, and areas of expertise have come together to offer their important and diverse perspectives in this edited book. This volume is a timely and welcome contribution to the literature on migration and health, one that specifically addresses the challenging questions of belonging, care, power, knowledge, and policy.

Catherine Panter-Brick is the Bruce A. and Davi-Ellen Chabner Professor of Anthropology, Health, and Global Affairs at Yale University. She is an expert on risk and resilience, having spent three decades working with people affected by war, poverty, and marginalization. A medical anthropologist, Panter-Brick was trained in both human biology and the social sciences. She has extensive experience leading mixed-methods research, having directed more than forty interdisciplinary projects in Afghanistan, Ethiopia, the Gambia, Jordan, Mexico, Nepal, Niger, Pakistan, Saudi Arabia, Tanzania, the UK, and the United States. For her work in humanitarian areas, she received the Lucy Mair Medal, awarded by the Royal Anthropology Institute to honor excellence in the application of anthropology to the active recognition of human dignity.

Introduction

Nadia El-Shaarawi and Stéphanie Larchanché

Migration is one of the defining issues of our time. The beginning of the twenty-first century has been characterized by a consistent increase in the number of people on the move and it seems that in nearly every year in recent memory, the United Nations reports a record increase in global migration. In 2020, for example, the UN reported that an estimated 281 million people around the world are international migrants (International Organization for Migration 2022). Yet such numbers do not provide us with the full scale of human mobility; excluded from this number are the hundreds of millions of people who migrate without crossing state borders, for reasons that include mobility for work or education, as well as fleeing from conflict, persecution, or environmental degradation, among others (International Organization for Migration 2020). As a dynamic and multifaceted process, migration affects individuals, families, communities, and societies across time and space in myriad ways. In this volume, we bring together anthropological scholarship that addresses one domain of these complex processes: the intersection of migration and health. In doing so, we seek to consider both migration and health from an inclusive, holistic, and critical perspective, undoing conventional ideas of the connection between these two vital topics and questioning some of the usual borders that are applied to both scholarly and public conversations on the topic. We ask: how is migration a health issue, and vice versa, how is health impacted by migration?

This edited volume explores, and challenges, the various borders of health and healthcare as they appear in the context of migration, while also unsettling some of the boundaries that structure conversations about human mobility and movement. The motif of challenging borders appears as powerfully evocative of contemporary migrants' experiences (Agier 2016), and we use it as a thread to help think through the challenges migrants face in attaining health and accessing healthcare as well as their efforts to transcend such boundaries. While readily construed as geographical and physical, borders can also be social, economic, political, historical, discursive, ideological, and disciplinary. These less visible borders may act more insidiously, as they constrain our thinking and inform scholarly policy and discursive responses to migration and migrants at different scales.

Despite the proliferation of scholarship on this topic, thematic, regional and sub-disciplinary boundaries have limited the extent to which the diverse anthropological perspectives on migration and health have come into conversation with one another. We argue that transcending such boundaries allows for a fruitful and more critical understanding of the intersections of migration and health, one which offers new ways of reckoning these two crucial topics both within, and beyond, academia. While the contributors to this book are all anthropologists, their work crosses subfields and addresses topics often not brought together. The work in this volume shares some anthropological hallmarks that we believe contribute to a rich understanding of the stakes of migration and health: long-term ethnographic fieldwork, locally situated analyses, and attention to the understandings and theorizations of our interlocutors, whether they are people on the move or health care providers. The contributors to this volume also draw on and contribute to what must, by definition, be a multidisciplinary conversation, as investigations of both migration and health draw on the expertise and experiences of scholars and practitioners in a wide range of fields. We hope this volume will be of interest not only to anthropologists, but to anyone interested in understanding the relationships between these two domains that are so vital to human life and its ability to flourish.

In this introduction, we begin by laying out our two key domains of interest, migration and health. Then we survey the landscape of contemporary global migration by describing current migration statistics and trends. We next discuss and, in the spirit of this volume, challenge the various categories used to describe migration and people who move. We complicate each of these categories, briefly discussing what they offer but also what they obscure. Next, we briefly survey the existing literature on the health effects of migration. We then turn to the larger theoretical motif of the volume, challenging borders. Finally, we describe the organization of the volume and review the contributions.

Thinking with Migration

As suggested by the subtitle of this book, our view of migration is expansive and transcends boundaries and categories that are often kept separate in scholarship, policy, and public debate. Indeed, there is no single, agreed-upon definition of the term "migration" or consensus about who is included in the category "migrant." Instead we see a proliferation of categories and terms used to define and describe people on the move; these terms structure how people are treated, often in violent and exclusionary ways. They also structure the terms of academic and public debates, which frequently end up mirroring and replicating these categories. To provide just one prominent example, despite the widely accepted critique that the separation between "refugees" and "migrants" does not represent the actual experiences and motivations of the people these categories describe, refugee studies and migration studies are often held apart as distinct fields, each with its own journals, conferences, and conversations. We argue that bringing together areas that are often kept siloed from one another creates fruitful possibilities for understanding the interlocking health effects of migration while also rendering visible significant differences that occur as a result of legal status, class, racialization, national identity, gender and sexual orientation, ability, and age, among others.

Counting and Classifying Migration

In order to trouble them later, we begin by sketching some of the existing ways of classifying and discussing migration. Broadly, migration refers to the movement of people from at least one place to another. But this general category encompasses a great diversity of experiences, practices, actors, institutions, and policies, each with different implications for questions of health and well-being. For example, the temporality of migration is one important dimension of comparison. People may move from one location to another and plan to stay permanently, or move for a temporary period, or travel seasonally between one or several locations, often for work. Journeys may take hours or years and may include multiple legs of travel as well as periods of waiting or transit that themselves can last years in some cases. The directionality of mobility is also variable. We often imagine migration to be linear and move in one direction, but it can also be circuitous, circular, or bi-directional. People may cross state borders, but, as mentioned above, most migration occurs within the borders of states. Who travels also varies: individuals, families of various configurations, and larger collectivities all migrate. The term "migrant" is sometimes applied to people who do not actually migrate, for example the children of immigrants or stateless populations who have been denied the rights and recognition associated with citizenship.

In this introduction, we use the term "migrant" in an inclusive way, irrespective of legal or social status. While recognizing its limitations, we have chosen this term partly because it is the most expansive term available, able to encompass a range of legal statuses and experiences, and partly because we seek to contribute to its destigmatization. At times, when describing particular policies, and especially in this section, we refer to the legal and political categories by which migrants are categorized. Doing so creates a tension: we acknowledge how these categories are used to govern and divide migrants, positioning some as deserving (Willen 2012) while irregularizing or illegalizing others (Jansen, Celikates, and Bloois 2015; Coutin 2003; Ngai 2014). At the same time, the policies and categories, themselves historically and politically constituted (Hathaway 2007), come to shape the subjective experiences and social and political positioning of migrants, with important implications for their well-being. If we take the structural determinants of health into account, one might argue that migration policy is always already policy that affects health and well-being. Anthropological research has been instrumental in documenting how processes of classifying and categorizing migrants themselves can have deleterious effects for mental health and well-being, especially when such processes interpolate migrants as security threats or criminals (Haas 2012). It is therefore important to document, empirically, the role that such categorizations have in creating differential experiences and status for migrants without taking the categories as natural or given.

Mindful of this variation and complexity, we begin this section with a brief snapshot of global migration trends, while also introducing some of the principal challenges of counting and classifying human mobility. Human migration is an age-old phenomenon that stretches back to the earliest periods of history, but its scale and its impact have changed with globalization, especially the proliferation of technology that renders migration more accessible (and at times is weaponized to make it more difficult) and global inequities that alternately make migration more necessary and difficult for some and easier for others.

Today, we are also able to access more information on migration and displacement. It must be stated, however, that there are challenges to collecting data on global migration, and therefore these figures must be viewed with caution. For a number of reasons, statistics do not always accurately reflect migration, either at a global, national or local scale. First, a person's immigration status can be fluid and change quickly, depending on the circumstances and local legal/policy settings. For example, many international migrants who may be described as "undocumented" or "irregular" enter countries on valid visas and then stay in contravention of one or more visa conditions. Second, in contexts where migration is criminalized, people have incentives, often existential ones, to avoid being enumerated, since to be counted might put them at risk of deportation, detention, or other punishment. Third, there is tremendous variation in terms of which agencies or institutions are responsible for migration. States and international organizations have different immigration policies, definitions, and ways of collecting data on migration, all of which makes it difficult to establish a harmonized approach to documenting migration globally. At times, the under- or overestimation of migration is part of a political strategy on the part of politicians or governments.

With these cautions in mind, certain empirical trends provide a general picture of contemporary global migration. The population of international migrants—people who cross at least one state border regardless of the cause of their mobility—has increased but remains relatively stable as a proportion of the world's population, approximately one in every thirty people (International Organization for Migration 2020). Close to half are women (48 percent), and 14 percent are children, 164 million are classified as migrant workers, 25.9 million are refugees, 41.3 million are internally displaced persons, and 3.9 million are stateless persons (International Organization for Migration 2020). Most international migrants (74 percent) are of working age (twenty to sixty-four years old). Europe and Asia currently host the largest number of international migrants, followed by North America and Africa. The impact of international migration on population change varies from one region to another. For example, in Europe, where the rate of proportional population change is the slowest, international migrants can be said to have mitigated decreasing populations in many European countries where birth rates are declining. Meanwhile, in Africa, steady population growth was reduced by emigration from the continent to other countries.

In international and much national law, refugees, as a particular category of cross-border forced migrant, are classified separately from other international migrants. Under the 1951 Refugee Convention and its 1967 Protocol, refugees are people who have crossed international borders seeking protection because of persecution on the basis of either race, religion, nationality, political opinion, or their membership in a particular social group. In both Africa and Latin America, regional conventions have broadened the definition of a refugee to include people fleeing war or generalized violence. In all cases though, a person's ability to claim protection and legal status is dependent on the non-voluntary nature of their displacement. As people understood as outside of the territorial bounds of the nation-state, and therefore unable to make political claims on the state (Malkki 1992), they lack what Hannah Arendt has referred to as "the right to have rights" (Arendt 1986). While the Refugee Convention sought to address this imbalance and ideally provide temporary protection with the goal of eventual reincorporation of the refugee within a national community, in practice contemporary asylum falls seriously short of this ideal.

Internal migration or displacement, as mentioned above, occurs within state borders and accounts for the majority of global migration although it is usually less regulated and harder to quantify. While we do not often think of internal migration as involving border-crossing, it is important to recall the history of control and criminalization of migration within particular states, including in apartheid South Africa or the Soviet Union, for example (Light 2012). Rural to urban migration makes up the majority of internal migration and is also frequently for work and study. Indeed, many of the early anthropological studies of migration focused on exactly this kind of mobility (e.g., Feldman 1975; Mangin 1970). However, internal migration can also take place from urban to rural or suburban locations. Internal displacement occurs when people are forced to flee as a result of conflict, disasters, environmental degradation, or development projects, among other causes. The Internal Displacement Monitoring Centre estimated that, at the end of 2019, 50.8 million people were internally displaced. Most of these people (45.7 million) were displaced as a result of conflict, although a sizeable number (5.1 million) were displaced as a result of disasters (Internal Displacement Monitoring Centre 2020).

Of course, internal and international migrants are not discrete, separate categories of people and the internal-international dichotomy is one of the borders that this volume seeks to unsettle. People often become internally displaced before becoming refugees or after they attempt to return to the country from which they fled. Secondary migration—when immigrants or refugees voluntarily move from one location to another within a country—is also common. For example, when refugees are resettled to the United States, they are initially assigned to specific locations but then often move on to other cities and towns where they find greater economic opportunities, more affordable cost of living, or to join family or community (Besteman 2016; Ott 2011).

Statelessness represents another set of conditions and experiences that is not well-addressed by existing structures, policies, and institutions. By definition, stateless people are in a vulnerable situation, as they are not recognized as nationals by any state. Whether the condition occurs as a result of gaps in citizenship laws, the creation of new states, or systematic and violent mass denationalization of particular groups of people, stateless persons face obstacles in accessing basic services—such as education, employment, or health care—and can suffer discrimination, abuse, and marginalization. While stateless persons are not necessarily migrants, their vulnerability and lack of rights may lead them to migrate, internally or across borders, and often irregularly, given the significant obstacles they can face in accessing travel documents and regular migration pathways. As part of its statelessness mandate, the United Nations High Commissioner for Refugees (UNCHR) reported 4.2 million stateless persons globally in 2019 (UNHCR 2020), however, this number is likely to be a significant underestimate because fewer than half of all states report statelessness, including some of the countries known to have the largest stateless populations. A pressing example of a population facing contemporary statelessness is the situation of the Rohingya, many of whom are internally displaced within Rakhine State in Myanmar or have sought safety in Bangladesh. Bangladesh and Myanmar were the countries with the first and third largest populations of stateless persons, respectively, in 2018 (around 906,000 stateless persons in Bangladesh and 620,000 in Myanmar) (UNHCR 2019). The combined burdens of statelessness and displacement have significant impacts on the health of Rohingya people as well as their ability to access health care (Ahmed et al. 2018).

Shared Stakes, Divergent Experiences

The discursive framings of migration, especially how people on the move are categorized as deserving or undeserving of international protection, inclusion, and rights, shape how states and other actors respond and have significant effects for migrants' lived experiences (Holmes and Castañeda 2016; Yarris and Castañeda 2015). Migration that is variously described as illegal, undocumented, unauthorized, irregular, or even "mixed" is often, if not always, discursively positioned as "undeserving" of rights and assistance (Willen 2012). Yet even those people who are categorized as refugees or (especially) asylum-seekers are not immune from being understood as undeserving (Fassin 2005), untrustworthy (Daniel and Knudsen 1995), or threatening (Papastergiadis 2006).

Perhaps one of the most powerful—and troubling—categorizations shaping the politics of deservingness in migration links assumptions about choice and agency to questions of migrant deservingness. This distinction is enshrined in international law and reflected in much of the policy and public discourse surrounding migration. According to this categorization, forced migrants (refugees) are compelled to seek protection by violence and persecution, while "economic" migrants choose to move in pursuit of better livelihoods. In this volume, we follow Kristin Yarris and Heide Castañeda's (2015) powerful challenge to the dichotomy between "forced" and "voluntary" migration. Although they are often treated as such, neither of these categories can be cleanly mapped onto distinct populations, as Elizabeth Marino and Heather Lazrus illustrate in their chapter in this volume. The categories themselves emerge from particular legal, political, and economic histories and their application to specific populations changes over time and are often more reflective of contemporary geopolitics than they are to the actual lives of the people they describe (Coutin 2011; Horton 2004).

Migration is a result of a complex interplay of acute events and longstanding global processes, personal and familial aspirations, and structural inequalities. For example, protracted and new conflicts have led to record levels of displacement, both in terms of the number of refugees and asylum-seekers and internally displaced persons. The total number of persons internally displaced by conflict and violence has almost doubled since 2000 and has risen sharply since 2010. But it is climate and weather-related disasters that triggered the vast majority of all new displacements, such as storms, floods, and droughts. Climate change must thus be taken into account as a central factor in contemporary migrations (Faas et al. 2019; Hastrup and Olwig 2012), and it will continue to trigger major changes for human organization at large (Oliver-Smith and Hoffman 2019). Climate change and environmental disasters are not, as anthropologists have noted, exclusively natural phenomenon, but are shaped and exacerbated by human action and inaction. Vulnerable and marginalized populations typically bear the brunt of dispossession associated with environmental catastrophes and climate change. Underlying more acute causes, globally ever-deepening socioeconomic inequalities and environmental destruction associated with structural forces of neoliberal capitalism and imperialism underpin much of the impetus for migration.

Given the role of broad structural inequities in shaping migration, and its current prominence in local, national, and global politics, it seems clear that migration, if differentially experienced, is part of our shared human condition. This shared quality of migration remains true even though the majority of the world's population remains either unable or unwilling to migrate. However, debates about migration tend to tacitly assume that migration policy only affects people who move. In her recent book on mixed-status families in the United States, Heide Castañeda illustrates how the precarity and illegalization of one undocumented family member comes to have powerful effects on the lives of other relatives, including those who are citizens and permanent residents (Castañeda 2019). On a population level, migration affects all our lives, even those of people who "stay home": perhaps someone in their family migrates, or the food they eat is picked and packaged by migrant workers, or they join a solidarity initiative providing assistance to refugees, or they are affected by a virus that travels alongside business people from one side of the globe to another. To provide one example of the broader social and economic impacts of migration, consider how remittances—transfers of resources from migrants back to kin or home communities—not only affect the livelihoods of migrants' families but are a major source of global capital flow, infusing community and national economies (Cohen 2011). More negatively, we see how discrimination and criminalization of migrants does not only end up affecting migrants but bleeds over into other groups who are perceived to be associated with them (Ngai 2014). For example, the stigma that is levied on undocumented immigrants in the United States is not only applied to them but becomes part of the lived experience of Latinx people regardless of legal status (Chavez 2003, 2013; Willen 2007). One of our key claims in this volume is that migration and health cannot be separated from the health of broader publics more generally. Migration affects us all.

The shared stakes of migration are often obscured by the ways that migration is depicted as a "crisis." Crisis narratives are applied to migration more generally (De Genova 2017; Holmes and Castañeda 2016; Cabot 2015) but are often especially present in discussions of migration and health. Framing migration in terms of crisis portrays mobility as a problem and obscures historical continuities through an insistent focus on an urgent present. But migration is not new. People have always moved; in some ways it is a fundamental human experience. And yet, at different moments, in different places, and for different people, movement is experienced, understood, and governed in radically diverse ways. Paying attention to local variations, and the ways they articulate with transnational links, connections, and collaborations, help us to make sense of current processes of migration and their implications for health and well-being. And putting contemporary migration into historical perspective helps to provide context and grounding for understanding the present as well as to critically interrogate growing xenophobic rhetoric that seeks to stoke fears of "migrant invasion." Crisis discourse also obscures the transnational connections, many of them emerging from histories of colonization, conflict, and exploitation, that precipitate and shape much migration (Danewid 2017; Mayblin 2017).

Governing Migration

Contemporary migration politics and policies also often obscure the common stakes of migration in ways that muddy, not clarify, our understanding. For example, although countries in the Global South host the vast majority of people on the move, immigration and asylum policies in Europe and North America have grown increasingly restrictive. These restrictions have included the proliferation, offshoring, and militarization of borders, the erosion of international and national protections for asylum-seekers and refugees, increased migrant detention, the intensification of deportation and push backs, and the rolling back of entitlements and assistance even to migrants who have been granted legal status. In the United States, for example—which for decades remained the top refugee resettlement country—there was a significant decline in the number of refugees resettled in the country due to the Trump administration's efforts to virtually eliminate resettlement by substantially lowering the annual refugee admission numbers and implementing enhanced security screening for refugees from "high-risk" countries. In fact, since 2001, there have been several legal immigration reforms that represented migrants as potential "terrorists," just one especially troubling dimension of an overall shift in focus from human rights to security in the treatment of asylum seekers in the United States as well as in Europe (Abbas 2018; Boyle and Busse 2006; Watters 2007).

These restrictions have typically been accompanied by nationalist, xenophobic, and racist rhetoric that treats migrants with suspicion, if not as an outright threat. What Nicholas De Genova has described as the "deportation regime" does not just exclude people through processes of illegalization. Instead, it includes migrants in selective conditions of precarity that maintain their role as excludable, and therefore vulnerable, subjects (De Genova 2002). Such exclusionary responses also have their precedents in older policies and attitudes about migration, many of which, like xenophobic rhetoric today, conflate mobility with a range of threats, including the specter of disease. In the United States, historical examples include the Chinese Exclusion Acts of the 1880s and the mid twentieth-century internment of Japanese Americans. Many of these punitive policies, both historical and present day, have clear and documented health effects (W. D. Lopez et al. 2017). Even after return or deportation, migrants continue to experience ongoing health consequences of discrimination and criminalizing policy and practice. Whitney Duncan terms such cross-border, long-term health effects "transnational disorders" (Duncan 2015). The health effects, while clearly borne most directly by migrants, do not only affect the health and well-being of migrants but also larger communities. For example, during the COVID-19 pandemic, immigration raids violated quarantine orders, placing larger populations at risk (M. M. Lopez and Holmes 2020), while the deportation of migrants who were COVID-19 positive (many of whom were likely infected in immigration detention facilities) from the United States to other countries may have led to the additional, unnecessary spread of the disease (Kassie and Marcolini 2020).

Contrary to what media coverage may convey (Holmes and Castañeda 2016), not everyone wants or is able to come to Europe, North America, or Australia. Overall, South to South migration is just as common as migration between the Global South and the Global North. For example, the vast majority of refugees, around 85 percent, have sought refuge in lower- to middle-income countries (UNHCR 2020) and the same is true for most internally displaced persons (Internal Displacement Monitoring Centre 2020). Why some migratory movements are politicized and rise to the level of "global crisis" while others are relatively ignored is itself an empirical and political question anthropologists and other scholars might consider (Peutz 2019).

It is not hard to imagine that the co-occurrence of record migration numbers alongside the erosion of protections and rights for people on the move poses immense challenges. In 2018, the United Nations launched The Global Compact for Migration and The Global Compact on Refugees. Both non-binding compacts emerged from the New York Declaration for Refugees and Migrants, the outcome of a United Nations General Assembly-led Summit largely in response to the mass movements of people fleeing Syria and other countries and traveling to Europe in 2015–16. The Compact for Migration is the first such comprehensive document that aims to address a range of different kinds of migration in one international agreement. Its stated goals include encouraging international cooperation on migration, as well as the collection of migration data, so that migration trends and patterns may be better understood. Among its 23 objectives, the Compact intends "to mitigate the adverse drivers and structural factors that hinder people from building and maintaining sustainable livelihoods in their countries of origin" as well as to "reduce the risks and vulnerabilities migrants face at different stages of migration" (Global Compact for Migration 2018). The Compact on Refugees' stated objectives are to (1) ease the pressure on host countries; (2) enhance refugee self-reliance; (3) expand access to third-country solutions; (4) support conditions in countries of origin for return in safety and dignity. The Compacts aim to offer new global frameworks and relationships for governing migration. Some scholars see the Compact as a strong foundation from which to support migrant health and well-being (Devakumar et al. 2019). However, the Compacts have also been criticized by scholars and activists for failing to more clearly lay out state responsibilities, significantly center migrants' rights—especially the right to health—and thereby more strongly protect the health and well-being of people on the move (Bozorgmehr and Biddle 2018; Chimni 2018; Gunst et al. 2019).

Health and Well-Being in the Context of Migration

If migration is a challenge to define, health is similarly broad, potentially encompassing a wide range of states of being, practices, individuals, and institutions. Medical anthropology's general concerns with the social and cultural dimensions of health, illness, and healing systems can all be applied to the subject of migration. Perhaps the most obvious place to begin is with the effects of migration for the health of people who move. Such effects are not inherent to mobility but emerge in relation to the conditions in which people move, especially the structural vulnerabilities and violence people face both in transit and at their destinations.

The Health Effects of Migration

While some studies suggest that migrants may be healthier than non-migrants, possibly because those who are less healthy tend not to migrate (Wingate and Alexander 2006), the literature generally demonstrates that migrants experience poorer mental and physical health (self-reported and clinically documented) than non-migrants. Clearly, migrant populations are diverse, and the immigration journey, immigration status, and life conditions in host societies altogether have significant implications for migrants' health and access to health services.

Recent scholarship in medical anthropology has documented how the greatest challenges to migrants' health and well-being are most often determined by precarious social and economic conditions and an overall political context that casts them as outsiders, illegitimate, or threatening (see, for example Castañeda 2019; Chavez 2013; Larchanché 2020; Kline 2019; Willen 2019). For those who flee violence or persecution, their psychological or physical health may be threatened even before they leave home. Along the way, stricter and more militarized border controls, including in transit countries and destination points, have not reduced immigration flows, but instead created longer and more perilous migration routes, placing migrants at greater risk for ill health or even death (Albahari 2015; De León 2015). Those who end up stuck at borders, or who spend time in camps, or are imprisoned in detention centers are even more exposed to health risk (Griffiths 2013; Carney 2017; Steel et al. 2006; Werthern et al. 2018; Eonomopoulou et al. 2017). Even once, or if, migrants reach their destination, they frequently face obstacles, including stigma and racism, which may also have effects over their life course and into subsequent generations. On the other hand, migration can be salutary, allowing people opportunities to increase their standard of living, access needed medical care, healthier food, and other determinants of health for themselves and their children. More privileged migrants, with access to structural advantages, capital, and privileged documents, travel with less effort and enjoy easier integration at their destination points. Yet even in difficult migration circumstances, including experiences of conflict and displacement, people demonstrate tremendous strength, hope, and resilience (Panter-Brick 2014; Panter-Brick and Eggerman 2012).

Most significantly, anthropological studies of migrant health reveal the importance of the social, political, and economic production of distress and disease (Farmer 2004; Kleinman, Das, and Lock 1997; Singer and Baer 1995), as well as the structures and dynamics that produce particular patterns of access to health services and the quality of those services (Castañeda et al. 2015; Willen et al. 2017). These cumulative conditions of adversity that produce ill health among migrants are referred to as "structural violence" (Farmer 2004). From that perspective, it can be said that migrants are structurally vulnerable to ill health (Quesada, Hart, and Bourgois 2011). For example, the COVID-19 pandemic highlighted how migrants suffered from a host of adverse conditions that limited their ability to quarantine and made them particularly at risk for exposure to the virus, such as lack of insurance (Duncan and Horton 2020), precarious housing conditions in social housing or shelters (Du Loû 2020), or lack of basic hygiene in encampments and detention centers (Agier et al. 2020). There has also been an increase in racial discrimination and hate crimes against Chinese and other Asian migrants identified as "vectors" for the virus (Tisserand and Wang 2020; Huang and Liu 2020).

A central issue debated in the literature is the notion of the "right to health," which is related to the concept of deservingness that we discussed earlier in this introduction (Willen 2011; 2012; and Willen and Cook, chapter 1 of this volume). Indeed, the social construction of distinct migrant groups by dominant groups in receiving societies impacts both migrant health and management by local public health institutions (Briggs and Mantini-Briggs 2003; Chavez 2013; Quesada et al. 2011). Public discourse in receiving countries often emphasizes the drain on national resources (whether in the medical sector or other social services) generated by migrants (Goldade 2009; Ormond and Nah 2019 and see Nolan Kline's contribution, chapter 7 of this volume). Paradoxically, ill health has become one of the few legitimate paths to legal status, leading migrants to rely on their "suffering body" to make claims on the state (Ticktin 2011). For example, Didier Fassin and Estelle d'Halluin (2007) documented how asylum policies in France intrumentalize asylum seekers' body as their main evidence for testimonial truth.

More recent ethnographies have taken a critical look that brings attention to how both the lived experience and social context of migrants also shape chronic disease or work-related injuries (Mendenhall 2016; Flynn 2018; Quesada et al. 2011). In the context of migrant labor more specifically, ethnographies thus reveal a conceptualization of migrants as "disposable" (Stuesse 2016), as well as economic and legal systems that not only enforce but normalize such vulnerability (Benson 2011; De Genova 2002; Holmes 2013; Horton 2016). In addition, the mental health of migrants has drawn significant attention in anthropological research. Specific challenges experienced by migrants include communication difficulties because of language and cultural differences, acculturative stress, and obstacles related to employment, social status and integration. In the context of mental healthcare provision, challenges may be related to the cultural formulation of symptoms and diagnostic categories that negatively impact diagnosis and treatment. Recent ethnographies have particularly shed light on the mental health impacts of asylum policies (El-Shaarawi 2015; Haas 2017) and have been critical of the popularization of the PTSD category as individualizing trauma, narrowly focusing on pre-migration events, as well as downplaying or ignoring cultural, linguistic or sociopolitical contexts (Fassin and Rechtman 2009; Kirmayer, Kienzler et al. 2010; Young 1997).

Migration and Care

In addition to health status, migration raises complex and challenging questions of care and policy. Beyond moving across geographical borders, migrants also move across medical systems. Significant changes in risks to health and therapeutic options thus accompany migration, but vary in relation to features of migrant populations such as gender, ethnicity, class, and legal status (Sargent and Larchanché 2009: 346). Although access to health care is only one, if important, determinant of health, migration and health care also exist in multiple, complex relationships. Take, on the one hand, how states increasingly exclude migrants from health care policies and programs as part of a larger strategy of excluding migrants more generally. But on the other hand, medical tourism remains an important way that people with means travel, seeking better or experimental treatment. And, as Rania Sweis shows (chapter 6, this volume), sometimes it is the medical professionals themselves who travel. Although clearly patterned along lines of race, gender, nationality, and class, the relationships between migration and health cannot be assumed and require empirical investigation.

As highlighted above, the multiple forms of social inequalities that migrants must face create a risk environment that is rarely taken into account in public health and medicine (Castañeda et al. 2015). Rather, anthropologists have documented how clinicians often emphasize individual behavior and intrinsic characteristics that are imbued by the collective narrative on migrants as radically Other or as a risk group. For example, anthropologists have critically assessed the use of the concept of "culture" in relation to healthcare policy and provision, in the context of mental health in particular (Carpenter-Song, Schwallie, and Longhofer 2007). Notable critiques focus on the patient-therapist interaction, marginalizing of non-biomedical representations of mental health suffering, and methods of assessment that potentially lead to unnecessary clinical referrals and may impact therapeutic outcomes (Good et al. 2011; Larchanché 2020). As a response, some anthropologists engaged with mental health issues affecting migrant populations have proposed clinically relevant recommendations (Carpenter-Song et al. 2007; Kirmayer, Guzder, and Rousseau 2013; Kleinman and Benson 2006; Larchanché 2020), including a "structural competency" approach that engages medicine with stigma and inequality (Metzl and Hansen 2014).

Politics and Policies of Migration and Health

Finally, intersecting with both health status and care, policy has important implications for health. Most obviously this relates to questions of health policy directed specifically at migrants, such as whether or not immigrants have access to national health care services or the funding and implementation of health care initiatives in contexts of mass displacement. Such policies can positively or negatively affect the health not only of migrants but also of larger populations. For example, in the coronavirus pandemic, policies that restrict undocumented immigrants' access to health care potentially create pockets of infection that harm immigrant communities but also increase the risk of the spread of the virus to the population as a whole (Duncan and Horton 2020). But policies intended to govern migration can themselves have both intended and unintended health consequences. As Jason De León (2015) has illustrated on the US southwest border, policies ostensibly intended to deter migration by making travel dangerous and even deadly have instead led to increased illness, injury, and death. Similar trends have been documented in the Mediterranean, where Europe's efforts to dissuade migrants from making dangerous sea journeys only make those journeys more deadly (Andersson 2014a, 2014b; Albahari 2015).

Thus, many health challenges are also a function of policies, political discourse, and public attitudes toward migrants (Carballo and Mourtala 2005; Willen 2011). In that context, migration has often elicited discourses of illegitimacy (Fassin 2004), suspicion (Haas and Shuman 2019) or fear associated with migrants in relation to specific disease categories or social issues that produce anxiety and mistrust (Chavez 2013; Larchanché 2020). One realm in which migrants may be cast as threatening to the nation is reproductive health. Migrant fertility specifically is frequently contested in narratives of the nation-state (Chavez 2017; Goldade 2009; Sargent 2007; Castañeda 2008).

Among the threats identified in the public imagination, the most prominent appear related to infectious diseases, leading to the characterization of migrants in general as a "risk group." These generalizations about the prevalence of diseases such as tuberculosis or HIV/AIDS often ignore that the communities migrants are coming from, or settling in, are characterized by structural disadvantages such as poor nutrition, inadequate housing or overcrowding, low education levels, and limited access to health services, which facilitate the spread of infectious disease. Instead, discourses of blame rely on anthropological notions of culture that place responsibility for an epidemic onto victims, such as in the case of cholera in Venezuela (Briggs and Mantini-Briggs 2003). Ultimately, both geographical and symbolic border practices themselves create conditions of pathogenic communicability (Chuengsatiansup and Limsawart 2019; Mason 2012).

Challenging Borders

The study of migration and health has been constrained by what we term "epistemic borders"—boundaries that challenge our abilities to speak to one another across subfields and disciplines. Among the most central, and problematic, of these epistemic borders are distinctions between "deserving" and "undeserving" migrants that continue to pervade conversations about migration. Even our vocabulary and the ways that we classify people on the move legally and politically constrain us within these borders. Take, for example, the distinction between refugee and migrant, which we will return to below. While these terms themselves have and can be fruitful objects of study, and while they come to have significant meaning for the people to whom they are ascribed, they nonetheless have been subject to important critique (Yarris and Castañeda 2015; Casas-Cortes et al. 2015). This epistemic border then reflects the extent to which the literatures in refugee studies and migration studies often do not seem to speak to one another, despite having significant common interests. Other epistemic borders that this volume seeks to challenge include dichotomies between health and mental health/well-being as well as those that emerge between more experience-near approaches and those that focus on structural violence. Not only does this volume seek to document some experiences faced by those who cross borders and those who offer them care or seek to classify, document, and understand them, but we also hope to challenge the epistemic borders that may limit wide-ranging, holistic analyses of the health and well-being of people on the move. If the defining feature of borders is the way that they are selectively permeable, it is our goal to use this metaphor to exceed the limits of the categorical containers we have been offered by academic and policy debates to consider what might be possible if we transgress and transcend these borders. Among the questions asked by this volume are: How does migration affect health status? What do practices of migrant health care look like, and how are they implicated in regimes of control or practices of solidarity?

The anthropological study of borders and boundaries, an area of recent growth within the discipline, addresses the ways that borders and boundaries are implicated in our understanding of subjectivity, migration, nationalism, and state-making, as well as cross-ethnic or cross-national conflict and cooperation. Increasingly, border studies' contributions have not been limited to what happens at, across, and around borders themselves, but have importantly provided a lens into major global political, economic, and cultural changes. This increased attention emerges in a time when, far from receding in the face of globalization, borders have proliferated (Ticktin 2011). Not all migrants cross state borders, of course, and borders affect not only those who cross them but also populations who live around them, who themselves shape borders (Cole and Wolf 1974; Lauth Bacas and Kavanagh 2013; Reeves 2014). But people on the move are the populations who most challenge and cross borders, whether they are material, bureaucratic, or metaphorical. Fredrik Barth's (1969) observation that boundaries, not only that which they contain, should be of interest to anthropologists because of the different ways in which they are expressed, maintained, and validated by the people who move between and across them, laid a foundation for thinking about boundaries and borders as being important to the self-conceptualizations of people and communities. Borders, then, and the people who contest them, provide a lens for looking at some fundamental questions: How is inclusion and exclusion negotiated and challenged? What relationships exist between territory, mobility, state power, inclusion/exclusion, and health and well-being? What happens when we transgress the tightly guarded boundaries around our concepts and ideas?

In times of fear, uncertainty, and anxiety, such as those that characterize the contemporary world for many people (Larchanché 2020), borders between those who belong and those who do not often harden (Castañeda 2019; Willen 2019). If this is a dynamic that we see repeated across many different settings, people in each nation or group draw those lines differently and reflect their own histories and ideologies in the process. Race, ethnicity, and religion are common markers of difference, and social representations that have evolved around these categories—while shaped by historical context—often travel across time. Anxieties that stem from fear in the face of social change or difference are culturally shaped, and almost without us realizing it, they recurrently crystallize around people who are considered "other"—migrants and their children.

These invisible borders, as Gloria Anzaldúa writes, include not only the borders that define us and them, but also creates a borderland, "a vague and undetermined place, created by the emotional residue of an unnatural boundary" (Anzaldúa 1987: 3). It is in this space that those who do not hold power and do not fit the dominant mold—migrants, of course, but according to Anzaldúa, also racialized people, LGBTQ+ people, disabled people, and indigenous people—have learned to navigate multiple worlds, to travel across the open wound "where the Third world grates against the First and bleeds" (Anzaldúa 1987: 3). The concept of *borderland* also draws our attention to the ways that borders can no longer be conceptualized solely in terms of state politics or imagined as the archetypical line that bisects sovereign territories (Alvarez 2012). For the "wound that bleeds" may be found on the bodies of those who feel they do not belong, based on imposed boundaries that separate them from broader communities of inclusion.

Recent ethnographic scholarship has focused on borders as a project, practice, and process as opposed to as an object. Bordering is a "technique that classifies and reclassifies both places and persons and their relations" (Green 2013: 350). An approach that looks at borders as a process allows for the possibility of people engaging strategically with borders and being both displaced and emplaced. It also renders visible borders that occur within, not between, the territory of states. Wendy Vogt (2018), for example, describes "arterial borders" as the ways that states patrol, police, and surveil migrants within national territories. Another important strand of recent border scholarship focuses on borderlands and non-territorial borders, such as maritime borders and boundaries (Ballinger 2003; Albahari 2015; Klepp 2010), and has laid the groundwork for a more dynamic and varied understanding of borders. This has also involved more analytical attention to the meaning of borders themselves, as the changes in the form and functions of borders may be leading to, or stemming from, changes in the notions of what constitutes a border. Scholarship on borderlands recognizes that we do not sit on the frontier of a border line, but instead "we are situated increasingly in the midst of a ubiquitous and multiple border, which establishes unmediated contacts with virtually 'all parts' of the world" (Balibar 2004: 1–2). Borders then become not only places, but also practices.

Many of the contributions in this volume aim at revealing such intangible borders, how they shape common sense narratives on migration in various contexts, and how they impact various stakeholders—from politicians to community representatives and leaders, health professionals, and migrants themselves. When resorting to the analytic of the border, we were careful to reflect power relations while not reducing the reality of immigration to a narrative between oppressors and victims, and several contributions that document migrants' experience specifically upset this category of victimhood (see Walker and Oliveira, chapter 2, and Yarris chapter 8). Instead, we take inspiration from our interlocutors and aim to think and discuss across legal categories, domains of interest, and geographical space.

Organization of the Volume:

Part I: Challenging the Borders of Belonging travels through various national and cultural contexts to identify these less visible borders of belonging and exclusion, how they define healthcare legitimacy, and assess how the political affects the biological, and vice versa. Sarah Willen and Jennifer Cook's introductory chapter unveils how such intangible borders are construed around the notion of *deservingness*, which they operationalize in relation to health. They provide a framework of analysis that identifies the various stakeholders, contextual variables, and evaluative criteria undergirding conceptions of health-related deservingness. In doing so, they help unveil the moral assumptions and "taken-for-granted truths" that constitute a collective "common sense" and that orient responses to such questions as "Who has access to healthcare coverage?" or "Who can benefit from specialty medicine?" Willen and Cook engage this framework of analysis through three case studies in three different contexts, which powerfully illustrate the situationally specific and context-dependent determinants that define the borders of belonging, and hence health-related deservingness. Ultimately, the authors call for investigations of how migrants themselves conceptualize their own deservingness and identify, resist or challenge the borders of belonging in the community(ies) they live in. What are the health implications of these borders for migrants and their families?

This is precisely what Rebecca Walker and Elsa Oliveira explore in their ethnography of cross-border migrant women in Johannesburg, South Africa. Drawing on an arts-based creative story project, Walker and Oliveira share the experiences of women—almost all of them asylum seekers and single parents—and their sense of well-being. The authors come to the concept of well-being from a holistic perspective, that is, one that encompasses community and social well-being, physical well-being, and access to healthcare, career well-being, and financial well-being. They also challenge the traditional focus on migration and health that highlights vulnerability—especially in light of pre-migration experiences, and instead unveil the more insidious structural determinants that negatively impact women's attempt to "keep well" in their host society. Doing so, Walker and Oliveira reveal how women struggle to find a sense of belonging in a context where the collective narrative blames foreign-born nationals for the country's social ills. Such a public narrative translates into concrete forms of discrimination and abuse, leading women to struggle to "be seen"—that is, treated with dignity and respect. This is even true of the healthcare domain, which in theory these women should be able to access: there again, the collective common sense negatively imbues healthcare professionals' judgment, leading them to see migrant women as malingerers or as contagious bodies, undeserving of medical care. Despite multiple layers of adversity, migrant women find energy to challenge the borders of belonging, by resisting gendered and cultural norms in particular.

If the women Walker and Oliveira describe challenge categories of belonging and exclusion in their everyday lives and in the sphere of health care, Elizabeth Marino and Heather Lazrus's chapter powerfully illustrates another way that the concepts and categories we commonly use to describe migration can fail to capture the empirical realities of human mobility. Marino and Lazrus's chapter draws on fieldwork conducted in Shishmaref, Alaska, and Nanumea, Tuvalu. Both of these communities are among the first to be identified as future "climate refugees" because their homes are threatened by environmental disaster, specifically flooding. However, the risk of a devastating major flood turns out to be only one of the migratory pressures people in both Shishmaref and Nanumea must reckon with. As a result, migration cannot be easily separated between forced displacement and voluntary migration as risks, pressures, and opportunities intersect and interact on the ground. Marino and Lazrus demonstrate how, rather than being separable into discrete categories, migration represents complex decisions made by individuals, families, and communities as they navigate risk of environmental disaster, deteriorating infrastructure, and other economic and social pressures. They argue that, in order for responses to climate change, environmental disaster, and climate-induced migration to be successful, they must take the lived experiences of the people most vulnerable to environmental disaster and degradation, including how people themselves relate to their environments, the constraints and pressures that lead to displacement, and the choices people make about their residences, livelihoods, and mobilities.

The second part, *Challenging the Borders of Care*, looks at how migrants' health status and needs challenge the borders of biomedical care, and argues for global perspectives on health that link the biological to the social, the political, and the personal. It gathers various experiences that have crossed the aforementioned borders to propose disciplinary articulations between field data and health settings. In her chapter on the development and practice of ethnopsychiatry in Italy, Cristiana Giordano describes how a local intellectual tradition of analyzing the relationship between hegemonic and subaltern cultures has opened a space for political action that would involve subalterns. In the context of psychiatric care, this implied denouncing institutional, normative psychiatry, to bring the focus back onto patients' experience and needs. In the context of migration, this meant allowing for "alternative modalities of healing and suffering" in the clinical context. Ethnopsychiatrists thus accept negotiating the traditional borders of psychiatric care as they integrate patients' own interpretations and worldviews and they see this confrontation of explanatory models as constitutive of the act of care, rather than the strict labeling of symptoms. Meanwhile, this form of therapeutic process challenges the dynamics of othering that otherwise actively marginalizes migrants in the host society.

Interestingly, in France, where in theory access to healthcare is universal—and as such "presents no borders to the sick," a combination of economic precarity, legal challenges, and language obstacles in practice challenge this access for vulnerable migrants in many ways. In that context, Carolyn Sargent, Laurent Zelek, and Anne Festa look at the importance of local associations in offering advice and assistance to those needing treatment for serious chronic conditions such as cancer and diabetes. They focus on one such association, AC Santé, located in Seine-Saint-Denis—considered the most structurally vulnerable department in the Paris metropolitan area. They describe the association professionals' efforts to create health paths that trigger the intervention and collaboration of professionals from different categories to address vulnerable migrant patients' health needs. Through the creation of innovative tools such as the "social dialogue meeting" or the EPICES score, the association specifically addresses the social dimensions of illness that typically elude traditional health institutions. By anticipating the needs of patients at the intersection of the biological and the social, they challenge the traditional borders of biomedical care. Sargent, Zelek, and Festa illustrate the impact of these efforts at providing holistic care through two poignant vignettes. The authors' pluridisciplinary collaboration also highlights the combined relevance of anthropological research and associative field actors to better inform health professionals on vulnerable migrant patients' needs and on the necessary adjustments for their treatment.

Rania Sweis provides an original contribution on how the act of caring itself may be driven by a sense of national belonging in the context of humanitarian aid, specifically the provision of health care to refugees and other populations affected by war. By documenting the experience of Syrian-American doctors' intervention during the Syrian Civil War, she challenges the notion that it is primarily white American or European aid workers who do humanitarian work, unsettling the imaginary of humanitarian care that often dominates the literature and the media. In doing so, she also disturbs the traditional East-West or North-South border divide that typically defines the context of humanitarian aid and creates a hierarchy of humanitarians, beyond hierarchies of care. Sweis thus shows how, in Syria, it is in fact local doctors and Arab emigrants—not foreign doctors—who provide most humanitarian aid to Syrians. While these doctors place their universal, professional ethics of beneficence and medical neutrality first, they reveal that both their cultural knowledge and attachment to the place of conflict undergirds their commitment to intervening in the context of war. In conclusion, Sweis contends that identity strongly matters in shaping global humanitarianism and that documenting the "reasonings" of humanitarian workers in war-devastated zones such as Syrian is paramount to obtaining "new insights into the nature of violence and its effects on human lives."

Finally, in the third part, *Challenging Policy Borders*, we gather perspectives on how various types of policies act as borders that directly and indirectly impact migrant health and their access to health care. Nolan Kline looks at the United States and examines how both the healthcare and immigration systems have become increasingly financialized. Based on a rhetoric that conflates both economic concerns and racial difference, vulnerable immigrants such as undocumented individuals or refugees are considered a "public charge" burdening the nation. More disturbingly, this "public charge" rhetoric has recently translated into policies that challenge immigrants' access to residency and citizenship. As a result, it creates a climate of fear among immigrants themselves who refrain from applying for benefits such as food or healthcare assistance. The enforcement of immigration laws through the militarization of borders or through detention also has negative health consequences for immigrants. While benefiting the security businesses or private prison companies who are profiting from aggressive immigration laws, detention conditions are abusive and traumatizing for migrants. In particular, the strategic use of family separation creates inhumane situations for families, with long-lasting mental health consequences. This is also true of detained undocumented migrants who identify as LGBTQ+, who suffer mistreatment and harassment from staff and other detainees. As Kline contends, crime and punishment were established to control and deter the presence of economically and racially undesirable immigrants. Under the Trump administration, policy measures such as the "remain in Mexico policy" or the announced end of the temporary protected status (TPS) for those fleeing civil conflict or natural disaster legitimate these violent control practices. Conversely, Kline shows, legal residency and citizenship have become easily accessible for wealthy individuals who wish to invest in the US economy. There is a commodification of citizenship statuses which reinforces global inequalities. Altogether, the financialization of immigration and related healthcare conditions in the US are part of a neoliberal agenda that serves to create a "political economy of belonging."

From Kline's account, we may be tempted to conclude that anti-immigrant policies erect borders that further victimize migrants and deny them any form of agency as political subjects, leading to deteriorated health status. But as Kristin Yarris skillfully shows in her chapter, the lived experience of migrants in response to aggressive policies may be more complex—or at least it may take different shapes depending on the local context. In the US state of Oregon, where Yarris carries out ongoing ethnography on migration and policy responses,—specifically on the state's "Sanctuary" law—advocates mobilized state law to protect immigrant community members from the federal Immigration and Customs Enforcement (ICE) measures. In fact, when this state law was challenged during the 2018 general elections, on account of the same rhetoric described earlier by Kline and others in this volume—migrants are a public charge and that their presence leads to increased crime and insecurity—community members testifying against the violation of the state law were able to reassert their right to belonging. Interestingly, Yarris shows, they did so by positioning themselves as victims of ICE family separation interventions and using this narrative positionality as a way to assert their political agency. Through her retranscription of the poignant testimonies, Yarris describes how the public context of hearings makes violence visible, and formally acknowledges speakers' political subjectivity. Therefore, it legitimates the lived experience of state violence, as well as the experience of trauma. Indeed, the trauma of family separation is no longer abstract nor is it restricted to an event (that of detention and deportation) or to an individual. Rather, this trauma is shown to have long-lasting effects on subsequent generations and impacts the immigrant community as a whole. Yarris thus concludes that, while this narrative strategy could have been seen as reinforcing migrants' victimhood, ultimately it emphasized migrants' political subjectivity and their right to belong.

Nadia El-Shaarawi is an Assistant Professor of Global Studies at Colby College. She is a cultural and medical anthropologist who specializes in transnational forced migration, humanitarian intervention, and mental health in the Middle East and North Africa. Her current book project analyzes how, in the aftermath of the 2003 invasion and occupation, Iraqi refugees in Cairo, Egypt, negotiated uncertain conditions of protracted urban exile. In collaboration with Maple Razsa, Nadia is also working on *Insurgent Mobilities*, a collaborative ethnography of the Balkan Route.

Stéphanie Larchanché is the research, studies and professional training department director at Centre Minkowska in Paris. She is also a lecturer at Université de Paris and Sigmund Freud University. As a medical anthropologist and psychotherapist, her work focuses on migrants' access to healthcare – mental health services in particular. She lives in Saint Denis, France. She is the author of *Cultural Anxieties: Managing Migrant Suffering in France*.

References

Abbas, Mustafa. 2018. "Working as a Medical Doctor in the Calais Migrant Camp." *Medicine, Conflict and Survival* 34(2): 69–73.

Agier, Michel L. 2016. *Borderlands: Towards an Anthropology of the Cosmopolitan Condition.* Cambridge: Polity.

Agier, Michel, Louis Barda, Véronique Nahoum Grappe, Claire Rodier, and Nan Suel. 2020. "Personnes Migrantes En Centres de Rétention et Campements: Désencamper Pour Protéger" [Migrants in Detention Centers and Camps: Move them out to Protect Them].*De Facto* 18:10–18.

Ahmed, Bayes, Miriam Orcutt, Peter Sammonds, Rachel Burns, Rita Issa, Ibrahim Abubakar, and Delan Devakumar. 2018. "Humanitarian Disaster for Rohingya Refugees: Impending Natural Hazards and Worsening Public Health Crises." *The Lancet Global Health* 6(5): e487–88.

Albahari, Maurizio. 2015. *Crimes of Peace: Mediterranean Migrations at the World's Deadliest Border.* Philadelphia: University of Pennsylvania Press.

Alvarez, R. R. Jr. 2012. "Reconceptualizing the Space of the Mexico-US Borderline." In *A Companion to Border Studies*, 538–56. Oxford: Wiley-Blackwell.

Andersson, Ruben. 2014a. *Illegality, Inc.: Clandestine Migration and the Business of Bordering Europe*, vol. 28. Oakland: University of California Press. https://books.google.com/books?hl=en&lr=&id=pcfuAwAAQBAJ&oi=fnd&pg=PP1&dq=andersson+illegality+inc&ots=Sjib24Rm8G&sig=GeDrKx2zH5-1Uj1CW7ufs0t2A7g.

———. 2014b. "Time and the Migrant Other: European Border Controls and the Temporal Economics of Illegality." *American Anthropologist* 116(4): 795–809. https://doi.org/10.1111/aman.12148.

Anzaldúa, Gloria. 1987. *Borderlands/La Frontera.* San Francisco, CA: Aunt Lute Books.

Arendt, Hannah. 1986. *The Origins of Totalitarianism*. London: Andre Deutsch.
Balibar, Etienne. 2009. "Europe as Borderland." *Environment and Planning D : Society and Space* 27: 190–215.
Ballinger, Pamela. 2003. *History in Exile: Memory and Identity at the Borders of the Balkans.* Princeton, NJ: Princeton University Press.
Barth, Fredrik. 1969. *Ethnic Groups and Boundaries: The Social Organization of Culture Difference.* London: George Allen and Unwin.
Benson, Peter. 2011. *Tobacco Capitalism: Growers, Migrant Workers, and the Changing Face of a Global Industry.* Princeton, NJ: Princeton University Press.
Besteman, Catherine. 2016. *Making Refuge.* Durham, NC: Duke University Press.
Bozorgmehr, Kayvan, and Louise Biddle. 2018. *New UN Compact for Migration Falls Short on Health.* London: British Medical Journal Publishing Group.
Briggs, Charles L., and Clara Mantini-Briggs. 2003. *Stories in the Time of Cholera: Racial Profiling during a Medical Nightmare.* Los Angeles: University of California Press.
Boyle, Elizabeth Heger and Erika Busse. 2006. "Institutional Vulnerability and Opportunity: Immigration and America's "War on Terror."" *Law and Social Inquiry*, 31(4): 947–74.
Cabot, Heath. 2015. "Crisis and Continuity: A Critical Look at the 'European Refugee Crisis.'" *Allegra Lab.*
Carballo, Manuel, and Mboup Mourtala. 2005. "International Migration and Health." Global Commission on International Migration, Geneva, September 2005. Geneva: International Centre for Migration and Health.
Carney, Megan A. 2017. "Sickness in the Detention System: Syndemics of Mental Distress, Malnutrition, and Immigration Stigma in the United States." In *Stigma Syndemics: New Directions in Biosocial Health*, ed. S. Lerman, B. Ostrach, and M. Singer, 119–40. Lanham, MD: Lexington Press.
Carpenter-Song, Elizabeth A., Megan Nordquest Schwallie, and Jeffrey Longhofer. 2007. "Cultural Competence Reexamined: Critique and Directions for the Future." *Psychiatric Services* 58(10): 1362–65.
Casas-Cortes, Maribel, Sebastian Cobarrubias, Nicholas De Genova, Glenda Garelli, Giorgio Grappi, Charles Heller, Sabine Hess, Bernd Kasparek, Sandro Mezzadra, and Brett Neilson. 2015. "New Keywords: Migration and Borders." *Cultural Studies* 29(1): 55–87.
Castañeda, Heide. 2008. "Anxieties over 'Demographic Theft' and Undocumented Migrant Reproduction in Germany." *Medical Anthropology Quarterly* 22(4): 340–59.
———. 2019. *Borders of Belonging: Struggle and Solidarity in Mixed-Status Immigrant Families.* Stanford, CA: Stanford University Press.
Castañeda, Heide, Seth M. Holmes, Daniel S. Madrigal, Maria-Elena DeTrinidad Young, Naomi Beyeler, and James Quesada. 2015. "Immigration as a Social Determinant of Health." *Annual Review of Public Health* 36: 375–92.
Chavez, Leo. 2003. "Immigration and Medical Anthropology." In *American Arrivals: Anthropology Engages the New Immigration*, ed. Nancy Foner, 197–227. Santa Fe: School of American Research Press.
———. 2013. *The Latino Threat: Constructing Immigrants, Citizens, and the Nation*, 2nd ed. Stanford, CA: Stanford University Press.
———. 2017. *Anchor Babies and the Challenge of Birthright Citizenship.* Stanford, CA: Stanford University Press.
Chimni, Bhupinder S. 2018. "Global Compact on Refugees: One Step Forward, Two Steps Back." *International Journal of Refugee Law* 30(4): 630–34.

Chuengsatiansup, K., and W. Limsawart. 2019. "Tuberculosis in the Borderlands: Migrants, Microbes and More-than-Human Borders." *Palgrave Commun* 5(31). https://doi.org/10.1057/s41599-019-0239-4.

Cohen, Jeffrey H. 2011. "Migration, Remittances, and Household Strategies." *Annual Review of Anthropology* 40(1): 103–14. https://doi.org/10.1146/annurev-anthro-081309-145851.

Cole, John W., and Eric R. Wolf. 1974. *The Hidden Frontier: Ecology and Ethnicity in an Alpine Valley*. New York: Academic Press.

Coutin, Susan Bibler. 2003. *Legalizing Moves: Salvadoran Immigrants' Struggle for US Residency*. Ann Arbor: University of Michigan Press.

———. 2011. "Falling Outside: Excavating the History of Central American Asylum Seekers." *Law & Social Inquiry* 36(3): 569–96. https://doi.org/10.1111/j.1747-4469.2011.01243.x.

Danewid, Ida. 2017. "White Innocence in the Black Mediterranean: Hospitality and the Erasure of History." *Third World Quarterly* 38(7): 1,674–89. https://doi.org/10.1080/01436597.2017.1331123.

Daniel, E. Valentine, and John Chr. Knudsen. 1995. *Mistrusting Refugees*. Berkeley: University of California Press.

De Genova, Nicholas. 2002. "Migrant 'Illegality' and Deportability in Everyday Life." *Annual Review of Anthropology* 31: 419–47.

———, ed. 2017. *The Borders of "Europe": Autonomy of Migration, Tactics of Bordering*. Durham, NC: Duke University Press.

De León, Jason. 2015. *The Land of Open Graves: Living and Dying on the Migrant Trail*, vol. 36. Oakland: University of California Press.

Devakumar, Delan, Neal Russell, Lisa Murphy, Kolitha Wickramage, Susan M. Sawyer, and Ibrahim Abubakar. 2019. "Children and Adolescents on the Move: What Does the Global Compact for Migration Mean for Their Health?" *The Lancet Child & Adolescent Health* 3(2): 64–66.

Du Loû, Annabel Desgrées. 2020. "Être Confinée En Hôtel Social Ou En Centre d'hébergement d'urgence" [Being Confined at a Social Hotel or at an Emergency Housing Centre]. *De Facto* 18: 30–35.

Duncan, Whitney L. 2015. "Transnational Disorders: Returned Migrants at Oaxaca's Psychiatric Hospital." *Medical Anthropology Quarterly* 29(1): 24–41.

Duncan, Whitney L., and Sarah Horton. 2020. "Serious Challenges and Potential Solutions for Immigrant Health During COVID-19." *Health Affairs Blog*, 18 April. http://doi.org/10.1377/hblog20200416.887086.

El-Shaarawi, Nadia. 2015. "Living an Uncertain Future: Temporality, Uncertainty and Well-Being among Iraqi Refugees in Egypt." *Social Analysis* 59(1): 38–56.

Eonomopoulou, Assimoula, Androula Pavli, Panagiota Stasinopoulou, Lambros A. Giannopoulos, and Sotirios Tsiodras. 2017. "Migrant Screening: Lessons Learned from the Migrant Holding Level at the Greek–Turkish Borders." *Journal of Infection and Public Health* 10(2): 177–84. https://doi.org/10.1016/j.jiph.2016.04.012.

Faas, A. J., Roberto E. Barrios, Elizabeth K. Marino, and Julie K. Maldonado. 2019. "Disaster and Climate Change-Related Displacements and Resettlements." *The Angry Earth: Disaster in Anthropological Perspective*, ed. Anthony Oliver-Smith and Susanna Hoffman,185. London: Routledge.

Farmer, Paul. 2004. "An Anthropology of Structural Violence." *Current Anthropology* 45(3): 305–25. https://doi.org/10.1086/382250.

Fassin, Didier. 2004. "Social Illegitimacy as a Foundation of Health Inequality: How the Political Treatment of Immigrants Illuminates a French Paradox." In *Unhealthy Health Policy: A Critical Anthropological Examination*, ed. Arachu Castro and Merrill Singer, 203–14. Walnut Creek, CA: Alta Mira.

———. 2005. "Compassion and Repression: The Moral Economy of Immigration Policies in France." *Cultural Anthropology* 20(3): 362–87.

Fassin, Didier, and Estelle d'Halluin. 2007. "Critical Evidence: The Politics of Trauma in French Asylum Policies." *Ethos* 35(3): 300–29. https://doi.org/10.1525/eth.2007.35.3.300.

Fassin, Didier, and Richard Rechtman. 2009. *The Empire of Trauma: An Inquiry into the Condition of Victimhood*. Princeton, NJ: Princeton University Press.

Feldman, Kerry. 1975. "Squatter Migration Dynamics in Davao City, Philippines." *Urban Anthropology* 4(2): 123–44.

Flynn, Michael A. 2018. "Im/Migration, Work, and Health: Anthropology and the Occupational Health of Labor Im/Migrants." *Anthropology of Work Review* 39(2): 116–23.

Goldade, Kathryn. 2009. "'Health Is Hard Here' or 'Health for All'? The Politics of Blame, Gender, and Health Care for Undocumented Nicaraguan Migrants in Costa Rica." *Medical Anthropology Quarterly* 23(4): 483–503.

Good, Mary-Jo DelVecchio, Sarah S. Willen, Seth Donal Hannah, Ken Vickery, and Lawrence Taeseng Park. 2011. *Shattering Culture: American Medicine Responds to Cultural Diversity*. New York: Russell Sage Foundation.

Green, Sarah. 2013. "Borders and the Relocation of Europe." *Annual Review of Anthropology* 42(1): 345–61.

Griffiths, Melanie. 2013. "Living with Uncertainty: Indefinite Immigration Detention.'" *Journal of Legal Anthropology* 1(3): 263–86.

Gunst, M., K. Jarman, V. Yarwood, S. Rokadiya, L. Capsaskis, M. Orcutt, and A. Abbara. 2019. "Healthcare Access for Refugees in Greece: Challenges and Opportunities." *Health Policy* 123(9): 818–24.

Haas, Bridget M. 2012. "Suffering and the Struggle for Recognition: Lived Experiences of the U.S. Political Asylum Process." San Diego: University of California San Diego. http://escholarship.org/uc/item/7pd0w87k#page-483.

———. 2017. "Citizens-in-Waiting, Deportees-in-Waiting: Power, Temporality, and Suffering in the U.S. Asylum System." *Ethos* 45(1): 75–97. https://doi.org/10.1111/etho.12150.

Haas, Bridget M., and Amy Shuman, eds. 2019. *Technologies of Suspicion and the Ethics of Obligation in Political Asylum*. Athens: Ohio University Press.

Hastrup, Kirsten, and Karen Fog Olwig. 2012. *Climate Change and Human Mobility: Challenges to the Social Sciences*. Cambridge: Cambridge University Press.

Hathaway, J. C. 2007. "Forced Migration Studies: Could We Agree Just to 'Date'?" *Journal of Refugee Studies* 20(3): 349–69.

Holmes, Seth. 2013. *Fresh Fruit, Broken Bodies: Migrant Farmworkers in the United States*. Berkeley: University of California Press.

Holmes, Seth, and Heide Castañeda. 2016. "Representing the 'European Refugee Crisis' in Germany and Beyond: Deservingness and Difference, Life and Death." *American Ethnologist* 43(1): 12–24.

Horton, Sarah. 2004. "Different Subjects: The Health Care System's Participation in the Differential Construction of the Cultural Citizenship of Cuban Refugees and Mexican Immigrants." *Medical Anthropology Quarterly* 18(4): 472–89.

———. 2016. "Ghost Workers: The Implications of Governing Immigration through Crime for Migrant Workplaces." *Anthropology of Work Review* 37(1): 11–23.

Huang, Junjian, and Raymond Liu. 2020. "Xenophobia in America in the Age of Coronavirus and Beyond." *Journal of Vascular and Interventional Radiology* 31(7): 1187–88. https://doi.org/10.1016/j.jvir.2020.04.020.

Internal Displacement Monitoring Centre. 2020. "Global Report on Internal Displacement 2020." Retrieved 4 January 2021 from https://www.internal-displacement.org/global-report/grid2020/.

International Organization for Migration. 2021. "World Migration Report 2022," ed. M. McAuliffe and A. Triandafyllidou. Geneva: IOM. https://publications.iom.int/books/world-migration-report-2022

International Organization for Migration. 2020. "World Migration Report 2020," ed. M. McAuliffe and B. Khadria. Geneva: IOM. https://publications.iom.int/books/world-migration-report-2020.

Jansen, Yolande, Robin Celikates, and Joost de Bloois. 2015. *The Irregularization of Migration in Contemporary Europe: Detention, Deportation, Drowning.* London: Rowman & Littlefield.

Kassie, Emily, and Barbara Marcolini. 2020. "'It Was Like a Time Bomb': How ICE Helped Spread the Coronavirus." *The New York Times*, 10 July 2020. https://www.nytimes.com/2020/07/10/us/ice-coronavirus-deportation.html.

Kirmayer, Laurence J., Jaswant Guzder, and Cécile Rousseau. 2013. *Cultural Consultation: Encountering the Other in Mental Health Care.* New York: Springer.

Kirmayer, Laurence J., Hanna Kienzler, Ahdel Hamid Afana, and Duncan Pedersen. 2010. "Trauma and Disasters in Social and Cultural Context." In *Principles of Social Psychiatry*, ed. C. Morgan and D. Bhugra, 155–77. Hoboken, NJ: Wiley Blackwell.

Kleinman, Arthur, and Peter Benson. 2006. "Anthropology in the Clinic: The Cultural Competency Problem and How to Fix It." *PLoS Medicine* 3(10): e294. https://doi.org/10.1371/journal.pmed.0030294.

Kleinman, Arthur, Veena Das, and Margaret M. Lock. 1997. *Social Suffering.* Berkeley: University of California Press.

Klepp, Silja. 2010. "A Contested Asylum System: The European Union between Refugee Protection and Border Control in the Mediterranean Sea." *European Journal of Migration and Law* 12(1): 1–21.

Kline, Nolan. 2019. *Pathogenic Policing: Immigration Enforcement and Health in the US South.* Rutgers University Press.

Larchanché, Stéphanie. 2020. *Cultural Anxieties: Managing Migrant Suffering in France.* New Brunswick, NJ: Rutgers University Press.

Lauth Bacas, Jutta, and William Kavanagh. 2013. "Border Encounters: Asymmetry and Proximity at Europe's Frontiers." In *Border Encounters: Asymmetry and Proximity at Europe's Frontiers*, ed. Jutta Lauth Bacas and William Kavanagh, 1–22. New York: Berghahn Books.

Light, Matthew A. 2012. "What Does It Mean to Control Migration? Soviet Mobility Policies in Comparative Perspective." *Law & Social Inquiry* 37(2): 395–429.

Lopez, Miriam Magaña, and Seth M. Holmes. 2020. "Raids on Immigrant Communities During the Pandemic Threaten the Country's Public Health." *American Journal of Public Health* 110(7): 958–59. https://doi.org/10.2105/AJPH.2020.305704.

Lopez, William D., Daniel J. Kruger, Jorge Delva, Mikel Llanes, Charo Ledón, Adreanne Waller, Melanie Harner, et al. 2017. "Health Implications of an Immigration Raid: Findings from a Latino Community in the Midwestern United States." *Journal of Immigrant and Minority Health* 19(3): 702–8. https://doi.org/10.1007/s10903-016-0390-6.

Malkki, Liisa. 1992. "National Geographic: The Rooting of Peoples and the Territorialization of National Identity Among Scholars and Refugees." *Cultural Anthropology* 7(1): 24–44. https://doi.org/10.1525/can.1992.7.1.02a00030.

Mangin, W. 1970. *Peasants in Cities: Readings in the Anthropology of Urbanization*. Boston: Houghton Mifflin.

Mason, Katherine A. 2012. "Mobile Migrants, Mobile Germs: Migration, Contagion, and Boundary-Building in Shenzhen, China after SARS." *Medical Anthropology* 31(2): 113–31.

Mayblin, Lucy. 2017. *Asylum after Empire: Colonial Legacies in the Politics of Asylum Seeking*. Lanham, MD: Rowman & Littlefield Publishers.

Mendenhall, Emily. 2016. *Syndemic Suffering: Social Distress, Depression, and Diabetes Among Mexican Immigrant Women*, vol. 4. London: Routledge.

Metzl, Jonathan, and Helena Hansen. 2014. "Structural Competency: Theorizing a New Medical Engagement with Stigma and Inequality." *Social Science & Medicine* 103: 126–33.

Ngai, Mae M. 2014. *Impossible Subjects: Illegal Aliens and the Making of Modern America—Updated Edition*. Princeton, NJ: Princeton University Press.

Oliver-Smith, Anthony, and Susanna M. Hoffman. 2019. *The Angry Earth: Disaster in Anthropological Perspective*. London: Routledge.

Ormond, Meghann, and Alice M. Nah. 2019. "Risk Entrepreneurship and the Construction of Healthcare Deservingness for 'Desirable,' 'Acceptable' and 'Disposable' Migrants in Malaysia." *Journal of Ethnic and Migration Studies* 46(20): 4,282–4,302.

Ott, Eleanor. 2011. "Get up and Go: Refugee Resettlement and Secondary Migration in the USA." Geneva: UNHCR. https://www.unhcr.org/4e5f9a079.html.

Panter-Brick, Catherine. 2014. "Health, Risk, and Resilience: Interdisciplinary Concepts and Applications." *Annual Review of Anthropology* 43: 431–48.

Panter-Brick, Catherine, and Mark Eggerman. 2012. "Understanding Culture, Resilience, and Mental Health: The Production of Hope." In *The Social Ecology of Resilience*, ed. Michael Unger, 369–86. New York: Springer.

Papastergiadis, Nikos. 2006. "The Invasion Complex: The Abject Other and Spaces of Violence." *Geografiska Annaler: Series B, Human Geography* 88(4): 429–42.

Peutz, Nathalie. 2019. "Comment: The Importance of Listening." *American Ethnologist* 46(3): 276–77.

Quesada, James, Laurie Kain Hart, and Philippe Bourgois. 2011. "Structural Vulnerability and Health: Latino Migrant Laborers in the United States." *Medical Anthropology* 30(4): 339–62.

Reeves, Madeleine. 2014. *Border Work: Spatial Lives of the State in Rural Central Asia*. Ithaca, NY: Cornell University Press. http://ebookcentral.proquest.com/lib/colby/detail.action?docID=3138578.

Sargent, Carolyn. 2007. "When the Personal Is Political: Contested Reproductive Strategies among West African Migrants in France." In *Reproductive Disruptions: Gender, Technology, and Biopolitics in the New Millennium*, ed. Marcia Inhorn. New York: Berghahn Books.

Sargent, Carolyn, and Stéphanie Larchanché. 2009. "The Construction of 'Cultural Difference' and Its Therapeutic Significance in Immigrant Mental Health Services in France." *Culture, Medicine, and Psychiatry* 33(1): 2–20.

Singer, Merrill, and Hans Baer. 1995. *Critical Medical Anthropology*. Boca Raton: Routledge.

Steel, Zachary, Derrick Silove, Robert Brooks, Shakeh Momartin, Bushra Alzuhairi, and Ina Susljik. 2006. "Impact of Immigration Detention and Temporary Protection on the Mental Health of Refugees." *The British Journal of Psychiatry* 188(1): 58–64. https://doi.org/10.1192/bjp.bp.104.007864.

Stuesse, Angela. 2016. *Scratching out a Living: Latinos, Race, and Work in the Deep South*, vol. 38. Oakland: University of California Press.
Ticktin, Miriam. 2011. *Casualties of Care: Immigration and the Politics of Humanitarianism in France*. Oakland: University of California Press.
Tisserand, Chloé, and Simeng Wang. 2020. "Combattre l'épidémie de Stéréotypes et de Racisme: Une Urgence Sociétale En Temps de Covid-19" [Combating the Stereotyping and Racism Epidemic: A Societal Emergency in Times of Covid-19]. Désinfox Migrations. Institut Convergences Migrations.
United Nations. 2018. Global Compact for Safe, Orderly and Regular Migration. Resolution adopted by the General Assembly on 19 December 2018. Available at: https://migrationnetwork.un.org/sites/g/files/tmzbdl416/files/docs/gcm-n1845199.pdf
UNHCR. 2019. "UNHCR Global Trends 2018." Geneva: UNHCR. https://www.unhcr.org/5d08d7ee7.pdf.
———. 2020. "UNHCR Global Trends 2019." Geneva: UNHCR. https://www.unhcr.org/statistics/unhcrstats/5ee200e37/unhcr-global-trends-2019.html.
Vogt, Wendy A. 2018. *Lives in Transit: Violence and Intimacy on the Migrant Journey*. Oakland: University of California Press.
Watters, Charles. 2007. "Refugees at Europe's Borders: The Moral Economy of Care." *Transcultural Psychiatry*, 44(3): 394-417.
Werthern, Martha von, Katy Robjant, Z. Chui, R. Schon, Livia Ottisova, Claire Mason, and Corneille Katona. 2018. "The Impact of Immigration Detention on Mental Health: A Systematic Review." *BMC Psychiatry* 18(1): 382. https://doi.org/10.1186/s12888-018-1945-y.
Willen, Sarah S. 2007. "Toward a Critical Phenomenology of 'Illegality': State Power, Criminalization, and Abjectivity among Undocumented Migrant Workers in Tel Aviv, Israel." *International Migration* 45(3): 8–38. https://doi.org/10.1111/j.1468-2435.2007.00409.x.
———. 2011. "Do 'Illegal' Im/Migrants Have a Right to Health? Engaging Ethical Theory as Social Practice at a Tel Aviv Open Clinic." *Medical Anthropology Quarterly* 25(3): 303–30.
———. 2012. "Migration, 'Illegality,' and Health: Mapping Embodied Vulnerability and Debating Health-Related Deservingness." *Social Science & Medicine*, Part Special Issue: Migration, "Illegality", and Health: Mapping Embodied Vulnerability and Debating Health-Related Deservingness, 74(6): 805–11. https://doi.org/10.1016/j.socscimed.2011.10.041.
———. 2019. *Fighting for Dignity: Migrant Lives at Israel's Margins*. Philadelphia: University of Pennsylvania Press.
Willen, Sarah S., Michael Knipper, César E. Abadía-Barrero, and Nadav Davidovitch. 2017. "Syndemic Vulnerability and the Right to Health." *The Lancet* 389(10072): 964–77.
Wingate, Martha S., and Greg R. Alexander. 2006. "The Healthy Migrant Theory: Variations in Pregnancy Outcomes among US-Born Migrants." *Social Science & Medicine* 62(2): 491–98.
Yarris, Kristin, and Heide Castañeda. 2015. "Special Issue Discourses of Displacement and Deservingness: Interrogating Distinctions between 'Economic' and 'Forced' Migration." *International Migration* 53(3): 64–69. https://doi.org/10.1111/imig.12170.
Young, Allan. 1997. *The Harmony of Illusions: Inventing Post-Traumatic Stress Disorder*. Princeton, NJ: Princeton University Press.

PART I
Challenging the Borders of Belonging

Definitions of belonging and identity provide the foundations on which borders are erected and performed. As such, they provide the starting point for our epistemic inquiry.

This section asks:

Upon which criteria—moral, social, political, economic, ecological, biological—is belonging defined? How are the borders of belonging, and alternatively exclusion, performed, maintained, and transgressed? How do they condition migrants' health statuses and healthcare access?

Chapter 1 opens with a conceptual and analytical framework for examining a central and powerful concept that both derives from and consolidates the borders of belonging: the notion of deservingness. As the roots of deservingness are multiple and may be difficult to grasp, this section introduces concrete and various contexts that will help readers operationalize the concept and understand its relation to health and healthcare access.

Chapter 2 helps us capture the empirical reality of how borders of belonging and deservingness are enacted to limit migrants' healthcare access and explore to what extent these borders impact migrants' own feelings of entitlement. Moreover, the chapter unsettles traditional approaches to migration that categorize migrants as vulnerable and as the victims of powerful systemic pressures. Chapter 2 challenges this vision to instead demonstrate how migrants contest categories of belonging and exclusion in their everyday lives as well as in the sphere of healthcare.

Chapter 3 complicates migration categories and dynamics further, challenging the neat dichotomy between "forced displacement" and "voluntary migration" that emerges from more traditional understandings of migration. In the context of climate change-related disasters, the authors draw our attention to the multitude of factors and actors involved in human mobility decisions. Like other chapters in the section (and the volume overall), this chapter highlights the importance of delving into lived experiences so as to fully capture migration pressures at the systemic, community, and individual levels and to challenge categories of "victimhood" that obscure migrants' agency and ability to challenge borders of belonging and negotiate health risks.

1
Must the Tired and Poor "Stand on Their Own Two Feet"?
Tools for Analyzing How Migrants' Deservingness Is Reckoned

Sarah S. Willen and Jennifer Cook

> MARTIN: Would you also agree that Emma Lazarus's words etched on the Statue of Liberty—give me your tired, your poor—are also part of the American ethos?
>
> CUCCINELLI: They certainly are—give me your tired and your poor who can stand on their own two feet and who will not become a public charge. That plaque was put on the Statue of Liberty at almost the same time as the first public charge law was passed—very interesting timing.
>
> MARTIN: Although you mention—the American dream is built on this idea that this is a place where you can come and build . . .
>
> CUCCINELLI: It's part of it.
>
> MARTIN: . . . A life.
>
> CUCCINELLI: Yeah, it's part of it.

In late summer 2019, Ken Cuccinelli, acting director of the United States Citizenship and Immigration Service in the Trump Administration, decided on the fly to rewrite the iconic words of Emma Lazarus, etched onto the base of the Statue of Liberty, during an interview with National Public Radio host Rachel Martin.[1] Lazarus's poem, "The New Colossus," was written in 1883 as part of a campaign to raise funds for the statue's pedestal. The poem was moving, and the campaign successful. Nearly 150 years later, Cuccinelli's comments, offered in defense of the Trump administration proposal to deny a path to citizenship for legal immigrants who drew on public benefits, pervert the sonnet's fundamental thrust:

> Not like the brazen giant of Greek fame,
> With conquering limbs astride from land to land;
> Here at our sea-washed, sunset gates shall stand
> A mighty woman with a torch, whose flame
> Is the imprisoned lightning, and her name
> Mother of Exiles. From her beacon-hand
> Glows world-wide welcome; her mild eyes command
> The air-bridged harbor that twin cities frame.
> "Keep, ancient lands, your storied pomp!" cries she
> With silent lips. "Give me your tired, your poor,
> Your huddled masses yearning to breathe free,
> The wretched refuse of your teeming shore.
> Send these, the homeless, tempest-tost to me,
> I lift my lamp beside the golden door!"

For Lazarus and those who helped fund the "beacon-hand" of "imprisoned lightning" that "glows world-wide welcome," migrants' yearning required little explanation. For this "Mother of Exiles," all seeking refuge deserve entry through the United States' "golden door." Cuccinelli, however, along with the administration he served and the voters who put Trump in the White House, saw things otherwise. From their standpoint, only immigrants who can support themselves financially are deserving of US beneficence. He viewed this not as a reinterpretation, let alone a gross misconstrual, of the historic symbolism of the Statue of Liberty and "The New Colossus." Rather, Cuccinelli claimed his interpretation—and not the more capacious interpretation circulating globally in art, media, and politics for well over a century—reflected the genuine "American ethos."

He is, of course, wrong, but that is not the point of this chapter. Rather, the aim is to show that social scientists' capacity to understand—and intervene in—debates about migration and, in particular, about migrants' health will depend on our ability to identify, uncover, and analyze the values and presumptions they entail: our ability, in other words, to understand how deservingness is reckoned by local actors with their own particular values, commitments, and agendas. To this end, we operationalize the concept of health-related deservingness (see Willen 2012a, 2012b) and illuminate its significance in debates about migration[2] and health in diverse settings and at multiple levels of analysis (Holmes et al. 2021; Viladrich 2019; Snell-Rood and Carpenter-Song 2018; Bourgois et al. 2017).

The significance of this task could not be starker or clearer than it is now, as this volume goes to press with a global pandemic raging around us. Think, for instance, of the many migrants to the United States, many of whom Cucinelli would have spurned, who were quickly re-moralized in spring 2020 as "essential workers." In the US economy, certain high-paid, high-status roles have long been viewed as more or less unquestionably "essential" to society's functioning—physicians, for instance. But in pandemic times, the calculus shifted, and a vast new cadre of "essential workers" was quickly re-appraised, among them hospital custodians and nursing home staff, delivery workers, farm workers, and food production workers—many of them low-paid, low-status, often racialized, and frequently migrants. Neither the nature of their work nor its intrinsic importance changed when the pandemic struck the United States in early 2020. Yet on a moment's notice, these newly "essential" migrant workers were suddenly recast as valued, and deserving—but deserving of what? Of brief spates of Friday evening pot-banging praise—or safe working conditions, adequate personal protective equipment included? Of laudatory media coverage—or of residency permits, citizenship, or a living wage, including retirement benefits and health insurance?

In this chapter, we contribute to the book's goal of challenging borders of belonging, policy, and care by exploring how such shifting "moral grammars and vocabularies" (Streinzer and Tošić forthcoming) are used to situate, and resituate, different migrants and migrant groups within sociomoral space. How, we ask, do such grammars and vocabularies emerge and become settled as hegemonic forms of common sense? How, after becoming stabilized in ideological and discursive regimes, might such grammars and vocabularies become unsettled, transformed, perhaps even inverted? How are such moral regimes experienced, sensed, and embodied—and how do they affect migrants' health and well-being? These are among the questions we ask.

We begin by considering how the notion of deservingness has been conceptualized in recent social science scholarship, where migrants comprise but one among many groups whose deservingness regularly comes into question. We then offer a framework for analyzing deservingness debates, with a particular focus on debates involving migrants' health. The framework involves three core elements: the *stakeholders* involved, the *contexts* in which such debates take place, and the *evaluative criteria* employed. In the final section, we put this framework into action by analyzing health-related deservingness debates in three migration settings: one in North America, one in Western Europe, and a third in the Middle East. Overall, we aim to provide strong scaffolding for broad-ranging, interdisciplinary inquiry into both how health-related deservingness is reckoned and how local deservingness assessments can affect the health of individuals and the communities in which they live.

Conceptualizing Deservingness

In an important sense, deservingness can be understood as the flip-side of rights. Whereas rights claims are expressed in a formal *juridical* discourse that presumes fundamental equality before the law, deservingness claims are articulated in a vernacular *moral* register that is situationally specific and context-dependent. Put differently, deservingness debates often have less to do with empirical evidence than with competing everyday responses to normative questions.

These vernacular responses generally mix subjective attitudes and presumptions with taken-for-granted truths regarded as collective "common sense." For instance, a debate might revolve around the question of "Who should have access to this particular healthcare service?" or "Should this person receive financial support in accessing this service?" In COVID times, debates rage around precisely such questions of resource allocation, including the allocation of vaccines. In many instances, the vernacular reasoning deployed in such debates is but loosely tethered to empirical realities. Often it carries a powerful emotional charge.

In a moment of public health crisis, normative and policy answers demand carefully reasoned answers. Yet in this chapter, as in this book, our aim is not normative but ethnographic. Our common project is an exercise in historically grounded critical scholarship—and it is also an attempt to nuance and complicate debates about migration and migrants' health that will become heightened as state, civil society, and individual stakeholders the world over grapple with the ethico-moral struggles that define this historical moment, among them the COVID-19 pandemic, the erosion of the post-World War II order, the imposition of austerity regimes, the arrival of large refugee populations from the Global South to Global North destinations, heightened climate concerns, and increasing pressure to confront the violent lives and afterlives of colonial conquest and racist domination.

Against this backdrop, we ask: How do rights claims and deservingness assessments differ? Both are social constructions (Schneider and Ingram 2005), but they diverge in key respects. First, unlike rights discourses, which presume blindness to individual particularities, deservingness assessments are *relational.* One assesses others' relative deservingness on the basis of two key factors: an implicit sense of one's own deservingness, and a sense of (actual or presumed) social connection to those whose deservingness is in question.

Second, deservingness assessments are *conditional* on presumed or actual features of those whose deservingness is in question—intrinsic or extrinsic, mutable or immutable—regardless of their salience. In short, rights are presumed to have universal significance, even when they are not universally enjoyed in practice, whereas deservingness is always reckoned in conditional terms.

Third, conceptions of deservingness are always grounded in a particular social and political *context.* Fourth, deservingness assessments are *syncretic*; they are simultaneously grounded in multiple sources of moral insight and experience. For instance, they may reflect an amalgamation of professional expertise, "common sense," and personal beliefs and experiences. Fifth, they are *infused with affect*, or emotion. Sixth, they are *mutable*; they are liable to shift and change in response to new knowledge and evolving circumstances. Finally—and perhaps self-evidently—deservingness assessments are *implicit*, unspoken, invisible.

In short, vernacular ways of reckoning deservingness in general, and health-related deservingness in particular, involve complex forms of moral reasoning. The impact of such assessments is neither arcane nor trivial. At the local and national levels, questions of "who deserves what" are pivotal, if implicit, throughout the political process. They shape the discourse and practice of legislators and policymakers (Chock 1991; Guetzkow 2010; Heyman 1998), bureaucrats and social workers responsible for the distribution of social welfare benefits (Blomberg et al. 2017; de Wilde 2017; van Oorschot et al. 2017; Fassin 2012), healthcare institutions (Horton 2004; Wailoo, Livingston, and Guarnaccia 2006), clinicians (Holmes 2012; Marrow 2011; Vanthuyne et al. 2013; Huschke 2014), the media (Yoo 2002, 2008), and ordinary citizens (Gilens 1999; Katz 1989; Will 1993). At an international level, such questions challenge us to confront the profound health implications of contemporary patterns of global inequality.

Deservingness and Welfare

Although the impact and salience of vernacular deservingness assessments are garnering attention in multiple fields, the most robust body of research on deservingness to date continues to take welfare as its focus. Some social scientists have sought to operationalize deservingness in terms of measurable variables or normative criteria (Appelbaum 2001; Appelbaum, Lennon, and Aber 2003; de Swaan 1988; Feather 1999; van Oorschot 2000, 2006). Others have explored the impact of recipient characteristics like racial or ethnic background (Gilens 1999; Guetzkow 2010; Horton 2004; Kootstra 2016; Morgen and Maskovsky 2003; Yoo 2008); the social positioning, demographic characteristics, or emotional state of deservingness "evaluators" (Olsen et al. 2003; Verkuyten 2004); level of responsibility for, or degree of control over, the circumstances producing a need for support (Appelbaum 2001; Appelbaum et al. 2003; de Swaan 1988; van Oorschot 2000; Will 1993; Scott 2008); and real or presumed associations with criminality (Morgen and Maskovsky 2003; Olsen et al. 2003) on deservingness assessments. Other scholars have examined the impact of context, including economic factors such as unemployment levels (Blekesaune and Quadagno 2003) as well as national and personal ideological frameworks (van Oorschot 2000). Additional avenues of inquiry include the impact of neoliberal influences on welfare and healthcare policy and practice (Bambra and Smith 2010; Guetzkow 2010; Horton 2004; Rylko-Bauer and Farmer 2002) and the impact of the media on public perception (Gollust, Lantz, and Ubel 2010; Lepianka 2017; van Oorschot et al. 2017; Van Doorn and Bos 2017; Viladrich 2019). Still other influential studies examine how constructions of "undeservingness" ignore structural inequalities and reproduce negative, often racialized stereotypes (Gilens 1999; Katz 1989; Yoo 2008). In general, deservingness assessments seem to vary based on perceptions of social proximity between the subjects of debate and those rendering their evaluations (Grove and Zwi 2006; Newton 2005).

Newer areas of inquiry include the role of implicit attitudes (de Vries 2017) and incorrect beliefs on deservingness perceptions (Bamberg Geiger 2017) and deservingness assessments of the rich (Ragusa 2017; Sadin 2017). Finally, an important new area of inquiry among both quantitative and qualitative social scientists involves the impact of sociopolitical changes—including mass migration, the spread of neoliberal ideas of responsible subjecthood, and the imposition of austerity policies in the wake of economic crisis (Roosma and Jeene 2017; Tošić and Streinzer forthcoming).

Health-Related Deservingness

In contrast to this robust welfare literature, the question of how deservingness is reckoned in the health domain is a relatively new domain of inquiry (see Gollust and Lynch 2010; Gollust et al. 2010; Lynch and Gollust 2010; Scott 2008). This is a complex matter of great significance, especially in an era of neoliberal pressures toward healthcare privatization and commoditization, soaring healthcare costs, growing health disparities both within countries and between rich and poor regions, and massive waves of unregulated migration over land and sea. In countries with historically strong commitments to universal healthcare and social service protections, existing rights and entitlements are increasingly imperiled (Larchanché 2012).

Important research questions abound: how do divergent stakeholders—the privileged and the disadvantaged, policymakers and voters, clinicians and patients—reckon health-related deservingness? What criteria influence deservingness assessments, and what role does ideology play? Who is responsible for providing healthcare, and how should costs be covered? How do moral questions of deservingness intersect with juridical questions of rights? How do they relate to questions of "fairness" (Daniels 2008; Lynch and Gollust 2010)? When are inclusive deservingness assessments purely aspirational, and when are they grounded in precedent, policy, or law?

In pursuing these questions, it is important to remember that health involves far more than just the presence or absence of disease or injury—and, moreover, more than just access to curative care. Equally important, if not more so, are the social determinants of good health: the upstream factors and structural conditions that predispose certain individuals and communities to be healthy in the first place (WHO Commission on Social Determinants of Health 2008). For example, given the "structural vulnerability" (Quesada, Hart, and Bourgois 2011) many migrants endure, their access to social determinants may be as limited as their access to curative care (Castañeda et al. 2015). Even under the best of circumstances, structural vulnerability renders many migrants more vulnerable, and less capable of addressing their health needs than their citizen counterparts (Carruth et al., 2021). This is especially true during the COVID-19 epidemic, as mobile and migrant populations—and especially those racialized to their discursive and ideological detriment—face heightened rates not only of exposure to the novel coronavirus, but also of dying as a result (Bowleg 2020; Devakumar et al. 2020; Gee et al. 2020; Hardeman et al. 2020; Maness et al. 2020; Orcutt et al. 2020). Failure to recognize these interlocking forms of disadvantage can perpetuate the tacit politics of blame that lead many stakeholders to deem migrants undeserving.

Not surprisingly, migrant health has become a central theme in the emerging literature on health-related deservingness. Scholars have asked, for instance: how do local and national policies, especially in the domains of immigration and health, affect local conceptions of deservingness (Marrow 2011; Marrow and Joseph 2015; Haas 2017; Kline 2019; Oliverio-Lauderdale 2014)? How do healthcare professionals' unspoken moral assumptions about their migrant patients influence clinical interactions (Holmes 2012; Larchanché 2012, 2020; Marrow 2011; Vanthuyne et al.

2013)? How do migrant health advocates deploy notions of human rights, humanitarianism, and other "idioms of social justice mobilization" (Willen 2011) in claiming migrants' deservingness, and with what effect (Gottlieb, Filc, and Davidovitch 2012; Tiedje and Plevak 2014)? How is migrants' deservingness framed, and contested, in public health literature (Viladrich 2012), or by supranational organizations like UNHCR (el-Shaarawi 2021)? And what about migrants' perspectives? Do different migrant groups regard themselves as deserving of access to healthcare, or of the social determinants of good health? How do others' negative assessments affect their lived experience (Chavez 2012; Larchanché 2012)? These are all crucial questions that demand further inquiry.

Health-Related Deservingness: A Framework for Analysis

Deservingness debates involve conversations, either in public or behind closed doors, in which divergent stakeholders express or enact competing views about whether a particular person or social group deserves a certain kind of attention, investment, or care. Although professional considerations and empirical evidence may play a role, such debates frequently hinge on vernacular assumptions that rely less on empirical evidence than "common-sense" knowledge and subjective moral commitments. Despite the pivotal role such assumptions play and their tangible effects, they tend to remain unspoken and implicit.

Elsewhere we have proposed that these vernacular forms of moral reasoning urgently require investigation—from multiple stakeholder and disciplinary perspectives, in different contexts and professional settings, and using a range of research methods (Willen 2012a). We develop this argument below. Our project is framed not by normative *philosophical* questions—for instance, about health and distributive justice—but rather by empirical *social scientific* questions: how are moral assessments and ethical decisions made in everyday social contexts? How do they find expression in particular forms of discourse and social practice? What sort of consequences do they effect?

Below we offer a model for investigating how different forms of vernacular moral reasoning inform local conversations about the kinds of health-related attention, investment, and care migrants do or do not deserve, and on what grounds. To parse the assumptions implicated in such debates, three key considerations demand attention: the range of relevant *stakeholders*, the multiple layers of *context* in which debates unfold, and the *evaluative criteria* stakeholders employ.

Stakeholders

The array of *stakeholders* engaged in local deservingness debates varies depending on the migrant group involved, the health resource in question, the domain in which a point of tension or contention arises, and the personal stakes for individual stakeholders. These may include policymakers (elected and appointed), politicians, the media (journalists, pundits, etc.), advocacy groups, and members of the broader public in their capacities as citizens, voters, and media consumers. In the health domain, other key stakeholders include not just healthcare providers (physicians, nurses, allied health professionals, etc.), but also public health professionals, clinical office staff, insurance administrators, and other "street level bureaucrats" (Lipsky 1980) who serve important gatekeeping functions. Ethicists, including bioethicists and public health ethicists, may be stakeholders as well. Migrants are, of course, key stakeholders in all such debates. Yet their voices often are muted—or, more egregiously, ignored.

Although professional considerations influence many stakeholders' views, subjective commitments play a crucial role as well. Politicians, for instance, are elected to represent their constituents, but their own moral values—and concern for their political futures—also play a role. Public health workers hold core professional commitments (e.g., to make wise use of public resources, to follow scientific best practices), but also face political considerations and personal interests, some moral and some tactical (e.g., to protect one's professional credibility—or job security). In healthcare settings, administrative staff must juggle professional expectations, institutional mandates, and personal views. For example, if a hospital's chief financial officer insists on up-front payment from undocumented patients, administrators may take it upon themselves to subject all patients they suspect to be undocumented—in the US context, for instance, all patients with names that suggest Latinx heritage—to heightened scrutiny.

Clinicians, like administrators, also are beholden to professional, personal, and political commitments, but they are bound by ethical codes that impose additional obligations as well (e.g., the Hippocratic Oath). Advocates, activists, and private citizens are also important stakeholders in deservingness debates. They may be more open and explicit about their political and moral commitments than those acting in a professional role.

To date, scholarship on deservingness has tended to focus primarily on the views of relatively advantaged stakeholders—those with power, influence or, at the very least, public voice. This, we contend, is insufficient. Further research is need to investigate how deservingness is reckoned both in relation to and, furthermore, from the perspectives of those most directly affected: individuals and groups commonly represented as undeserving. Research on migrants' perspectives may reveal appreciable differences between their own ethical calculus and modes of moral reasoning, on one hand, and those of other, non-migrant stakeholders, on the other. Moreover, their views of their own and others' relative deservingness are likely to influence their care-seeking behavior as well as their overall health and well-being (see, for example, Larchanché 2012).

Context

Context is another key element in deservingness debates. Four contextual domains are especially significant: history, law, politics, and economics. Below we highlight a few considerations that arise in each, recognizing that these domains themselves overlap and entwine.

From a historical perspective, one might ask: how have past experiences—either negative (e.g., drought, famine, political turmoil, war) or positive (e.g., France's legacy as home of the *Droits de l'homme*)—influenced current views of migrants and migration? Does a particular locale have its own history as a "receiving" community, a "sending" community—or perhaps both at different times? Has it historically been welcoming or restrictive toward migrants? How do views of current migrant populations compare with attitudes toward earlier arrivals, and why?

The *legal* realm is extraordinarily complex in its own right. At the international level, to what relevant international treaties and conventions is a given country signatory, and how do those international commitments influence policymaking, advocacy efforts, and public opinion? At the national level, who is and is not permitted either to enter the country or to immigrate, and under what conditions? How does national migration law influence public opinion regarding newcomers' opportunities, or lack of opportunities, for membership and social inclusion? How have migration laws changed over time?

The impact of political and economic context on local deservingness debates cannot be underestimated. In the *political* realm, to what degree is migration a local concern, and in what respects? What role do political ideologies and other value systems (e.g., religion) play in framing local debate? How do such commitments inform the views of influential political parties? Vocal minorities? The courts? Advocacy and activist groups? Do migrants themselves play an active role in local political conversation? If not, what impedes their participation?

In *economic* terms, how is the local economy performing, and what economic role do migrants play? Are they regarded as a boon or a threat to the local economy? As a valued source of labor, or unwelcome competitors for citizen-workers? The economic health of the local public health and clinical care systems also demands consideration. What health services can migrants access, and who foots the bill? Are these systems overburdened—or perceived to be—and if so, how are migrants' health needs conceptualized and discussed?

Evaluative Criteria

Finally, what *evaluative criteria* inform local debates about migrants' health-related deservingness? In reckoning migrants' relative deservingness, stakeholders often make presumptions about migrants' lives and life circumstances that mix collective "common sense," personal attitudes, and politicized forms of emotion. The connections between such presumptions and empirical realities may be tenuous at best. Wim van Oorschot (2000) suggests that five evaluative criteria, summarized with the acronym CARIN, inform deservingness assessments: control, attitude, reciprocity, identity, and need. Drawing inspiration from van Oorschot but taking migration as our specific focus, below we highlight five more specific considerations that shape local debates about who migrants are and what they do or do not deserve: migration motive, legal status, moral character, vulnerability, and social proximity to members of the broader society. Although these characteristics figure in general assessments of migrants' deservingness, they are especially salient in reckoning their deservingness of health-related attention, investment, or care.

Migration Motives

Migrants' presumed motives feature prominently in local deservingness debates. An especially bright line is assumed to distinguish "economic migrants" (who ostensibly left their country to pursue economic opportunity) from "forced migrants" (presumed to have fled violent conflict, political persecution, or natural disaster). Although this distinction is typically presented as clear-cut and self-evident, realities are considerably more complex (see, for example, Yarris and Castañeda 2015). For instance, asylum-seekers who have fled violence or oppression but fail to translate their experiences into bureaucratically legible categories will likely find their claims denied. Other migrants leave home fleeing poverty, including impoverishment resulting from climate change, only to find that their migration circumstances are not deemed worthy of recognition or status in their new countries of residence.

People tend to be viewed and treated in very different ways depending on their classification as either "economic" or "forced" migrants—categories that (often mistakenly) are presumed to be distinct. "Forced" migrants generally are represented as unfortunate, faultless victims of circumstance who deserve society's attention and material support. This logic is often invoked to mobilize humanitarian and human rights commitments at the national and international levels. "Economic" migrants, in contrast, are often assumed to have chosen freely to migrate and, on these grounds, are deemed responsible for their own fates.

This pattern of moral valuation can vary—for instance, when national policies themselves influence how particular groups' deservingness is reckoned. Policies that prohibit asylum-seekers from working while their petitions are pending, for example, force them to rely on interim government support. As a result, migrants who would otherwise be regarded as faultless and hence deserving victims may be reimagined as a burden to society (Sales 2002; Watters 2007).

Legal Status

Presumptions about migrants' legal status also figure centrally in local deservingness debates. Although the very notion of legal status would seem to hinge on a straightforward distinction, such matters often are far from clear-cut. Deservingness debates rarely account for this complex fluidity.

There is, of course, nothing natural or self-evident about legal statuses; they are human creations designed to meet political demands. They are also varied, amenable to change, and differentially enforced. A wide range of possible statuses exists both across migration settings and even within a single country. For instance, some residence visas permit study but forbid work, and some time-delimited work permits forbid permanent residence or family reunification. Migrants seeking asylum or refugee status may hold a temporary status valid only while their petitions are pending. And in countries that grant citizenship on the basis of *jus soli* (birthright citizenship), statuses may vary within a single household or family. Often, violating the terms of one's authorization can automatically trigger a loss of legal status and consequent slip into "illegality."

Yet legal status is more than just a juridical category. It is also morally charged, and different forms of status are imbued with different moral valences. Unauthorized border-crossing, for instance, may be seen as evidence of immorality—or, worse still, of criminality. In either case, presumptions about legal status powerfully influence stakeholder assessments.

Moral Character

Debates about health-related deservingness hinge on impressionistic judgments about multiple aspects of migrants' moral character. For instance, stakeholders may make presumptions about a migrant's or migrant community's economic productivity, personal responsibility, fulfillment of family obligations, and associations with criminality. Are migrants presumed to contribute to the economy, or to society, through their labor, whether skilled or unskilled? To pay taxes? To depend on welfare, social support, or government programs? Are they seen as willing to integrate into the broader society? On all of these counts, vernacular presumptions influence deservingness debates, even when they are contradicted by empirical evidence (Chauvin Garcés-Mascareñas, and Kraler 2013; Chauvin and Garcés-Mascareñas 2014).

The same holds true for family status. How are migrants' family configurations imagined in comparison to idealized notions of a "normal" family? Are parents viewed as more morally upstanding, and hence more deserving, than single adults? Mothers more deserving than fathers? Parents who live with their children more deserving than those who have entrusted their children to the care of extended family members?

The element of criminality is a complicated one, especially given the recent convergence of immigration enforcement efforts and criminal justice in what has been described as "crimmigration law" (Stumpf 2006). When migrants with precarious legal status engage in informal or illicit activities as a survival strategy (e.g., working or selling goods without a permit, using other people's identification documents, etc.), their actions may be interpreted as signs of immorality and hence undeservingness. Associations between migrants and criminality, even when spurious, are often bandied about with the explicit goal of inflaming xenophobic sentiment.

Vulnerability

Presumptions of vulnerability also figure prominently in deservingness debates. Migrants considered especially vulnerable may be more likely to draw sympathy and, as a result, may be regarded as more deserving than those viewed as less vulnerable.

Various criteria are used to gauge migrants' vulnerability including gender, sexual orientation, or sexual identity; physical or mental disability; past experiences of victimization (i.e., status as a survivor of violent crime, domestic violence, or sex trafficking); life stage; and health status. Certain individuals—for instance, women, children, the elderly, the severely ill, people with disabilities, and individuals with non-conforming gender or sexual identities—may be regarded as more vulnerable than other migrants and, on that basis, more deserving. Depending on local context and relevant stakeholders' views, however, certain migrants' claims of vulnerability may be deemed suspect—for instance, because they fail to conform to social norms, are perceived as attempts to "cheat the system," or bear some form of social stigma. Migrants living with HIV/AIDS, for example, may not be seen as deserving despite the severity of their disease due to irrational fears of disease transmission. Alternatively, stakeholders may question the morality of those afflicted by HIV/AIDS because of stereotypical associations, for instance, with homosexuality or promiscuity. The example of HIV reveals how evaluations of migrant morality and discussions of vulnerability can intersect in ways that affect deservingness assessments more broadly.

The relative visibility of one's source of vulnerability or affliction can also play a role in how deservingness is assessed. Sometimes a visible ailment (e.g., a missing limb from a landmine accident) is more likely to garner a sympathetic evaluation than a condition that is less visible (e.g., mental illness). As a result, migrants who have suffered often feel pressure, whether implicit or explicit, to bare their afflictions and "perform" vulnerability, even when doing so is embarrassing, humiliating, and/or contrary to their own sense of agency.

Social Proximity

Perceived social proximity between migrant populations and citizens is another key criterion in local deservingness debates. Proximity may be reckoned in terms of ostensibly intrinsic features (e.g., race/ethnicity, language, or religion) or extrinsic features (e.g., willingness to learn the local language, follow local gender norms, or otherwise endeavor to integrate into the broader society). Presumptions of social proximity generally lead migrants regarded as more "like us" to be deemed more deserving than others. On the other hand, in some contexts, stakeholders may invoke societal values like diversity or multiculturalism in an attempt to advocate for inclusiveness.

Assessments of social proximity are deeply influenced by local context. In relatively homogenous societies, for instance, racial, ethnic, religious, or cultural difference may be regarded as a threat to the collective. In countries with a long history of immigration, new migrants may be discursively aligned with older migrant groups with whom they share, or are presumed to share, key features. Aspects of local ideological, political, and historical context can influence perceptions of social proximity and heighten concern about particular groups (e.g., about migrants of color in majority white societies or about Muslim migrants in societies that are predominantly Christian).

Health-Related Deservingness: Three Debates

How do these forms of vernacular moral reasoning figure in localized debates about migrants' health-related deservingness? To address this question, we turn now to three cases: one from North America, one from Western Europe, and one from the Middle East. In discussing each case, we engage all elements of the framework introduced above (stakeholders, context, and evaluative criteria) while foregrounding one of the three. Each case provides a vivid illustration of how vernacular conceptions of health-related deservingness can be implicated in the domains of migrant health research, policy, or practice.

Organs for the Undocumented? A "Bungled Transplant" in the United States

In 2003, seventeen-year-old Jesica Santillan underwent a heart and lung transplant at Duke University Medical Center in Durham, North Carolina. Just after the surgery, routine post-operative blood tests revealed a terrible mistake: Santillan had received organs of an incompatible blood type. In a frantic effort to correct the error, her doctors procured another set of organs and performed a second transplant. Yet the damage was too great for her already weakened system, and she died several days later.

The story of the "bungled transplant" (Wailoo et al. 2006) made local and national headlines. How could such a mistake occur in one of the nation's premier medical institutions, the American public wanted to know. Who was to blame? As the media dug deeper into the details of the case, the tone of the conversation shifted, and spectators began asking a decidedly more contentious question: did Santillan even deserve a transplant in the first place?

From a clinical standpoint, physicians establish eligibility for organ transplantation using sophisticated biomedical algorithms. In Santillan's case, post-mortem eligibility debates revolved not around biology, but around biography—especially the fact that Santillan and her mother had entered the United States without legal authorization when she was thirteen. Commentators labeled Santillan an "illegal immigrant" and debated whether or not she deserved the medical care she had received. Some contended that only citizens should have access to "citizen organs" (Chavez 2006: 292) and declared Santillan and other "illegals" inherently undeserving. Others pointed to Santillan's youthful innocence and life-threatening illness as evidence of her deservingness. The tragedy of Jesica Santillan's death and ensuing controversy highlight an important but under-examined issue: the impact of vernacular deservingness assessments on broader debates about migration and health.

The tragedy of Santillan's death also spurred high-profile debate among an impassioned array of stakeholders. Should she have received a heart and lung transplant in the first place? After the botched transplant that led those organs to fail, should she have received a second? Pundits and the general public seized on her story as an opportunity to debate a broader set of questions. Should undocumented immigrants receive healthcare in the United States at all? If so, what kind of care ought they to receive, under what conditions, and with what limitations, if any? Finally, who should pay?

In Santillan's case, as in any deservingness debate, context matters. Despite the country's "melting pot" origin myth, the history of restrictive immigration policy and anti-immigrant sentiment in the United States runs deep (Ngai 2004). Especially in times of economic vulnerability, US public opinion has tended to portray migrants and immigrants, and unauthorized migrants in particular, as a drain on resources and a threat to national sovereignty (Chavez 2012; Portes, Fernández-Kelly, and Light 2012). When Santillan and her family moved to the largely agricultural southern state of North Carolina in 2003, a new wave of Latino migrants seeking agricultural work had just begun to arrive (Kochhar, Ruro, and Tafoya 2005). Although US citizens generally have been loath to take up jobs in the agricultural sector, fears of economic competition and cultural and demographic change have at times fueled xenophobic sentiment, especially in places like North Carolina, where Latino immigrants are a relatively new population (Marrow 2011).

A wide range of stakeholders participated in the stormy debates that erupted around Santillan's treatment and subsequent death, among them the two medical institutions involved in her care, the media, right-wing political pundits, and a white, middle-aged, local businessman named Mack Mahoney who first learned of Santillan's illness from the local newspaper. Compelled by her plight, Mahoney founded a charity to support her medical care and became the family's informal, if self-appointed, spokesman. In his public statements, Mahoney cited Santillan's youthful innocence as well as her frail, deteriorating body as evidence that she was a deserving candidate for transplant surgery. At times, he even infantilized her by describing her as a dying "baby" even though at seventeen she was nearly a legal adult (Wailoo et al. 2006: 304).

Following her death, a heated media debate focused on Santillan's unauthorized migration status. Conservative commentators leveraged her story to intervene politically in national conversations about immigration. Right-wing pundit Michelle Malkin, for instance, contended that Santillan symbolized a larger problem in the United States where "[t]he costs of illegal alien healthcare are crippling hospitals across the country" (Malkin 2003). In Michelle Malkin's narrative, Santillan was one of millions of "illegal aliens" flooding the country seeking access to already scarce resources.

Yet Malkin's account ignored several key facts. First, unlike most unauthorized migrants in the United States, Santillan's mother was covered by an employment-based private health insurance policy. Given the United States' employment-based insurance system, Santillan therefore was covered as her dependent. Additional costs were covered by private donations generated through Mahoney's charity.

Another conservative columnist, Joe Kovacs, compared Santillan to a different young woman awaiting a lung transplant, Lauren Averitt. According to Kovacs, Averitt—a desperately ill, law-abiding citizen—clearly was more deserving than Santillan. "[Il]legal aliens like Santillan," he wrote, "are able to leapfrog ahead of the many thousands of U.S. citizens patiently waiting and praying for their own personal miracle" (Kovacs 2003). From his standpoint, citizenship is more than a legal status; it is imbued with moral meaning—with life-or-death implications. Santillan's unauthorized border-crossing is portrayed as both criminal and immoral, as is her supposed desire and ability to jump ahead of US citizens on the transplant waiting list. In this account, Santillan herself is assigned culpability despite her youth and vulnerability, and even though her mother (and not she herself) initiated their migration.

The institutional stakeholders, Duke Medical Center and the United Network for Organ Sharing (UNOS), took a markedly different tactic. In their official responses, neither addressed Santillan's legal status. Each issued a carefully worded public statement in a cool, professional tone that contrasted sharply with the heated media fervor. Duke's response was particularly measured, likely due to concerns about legal liability for Santillan's death.

Much can be learned from this case about how migrants' health-related deservingness is reckoned. Above all, the contentious conversation following Santillan's death reveals just how low the threshold can be for involvement as a stakeholder—and, moreover, how quickly a relatively distant set of stakeholders can turn a localized discussion about a particular individual's health needs into a lightning rod for much broader public debate.

Not Sick Enough: Illness, Vulnerability, and Deservingness in Western Europe

In 2008, a very different deservingness debate unfolded in the United Kingdom about Ama Sumani,[3] a thirty-nine-year-old woman of Ghanaian origin and mother of two who was ordered removed from the UK despite the fact that she was undergoing life-saving treatment for malignant myeloma, a deadly form of cancer (Lawrance 2012). At that time seriously ill migrants ordered to leave the country could seek relief from removal[4] through appeal under Article 3 of the European Convention on Human Rights, which prohibits any action that would constitute "inhuman treatment" (Council of Europe 1950). Decisions regarding humanitarian relief under Article 3 are made by an immigration judge on a case-by-case basis. Sumani appealed her removal decision and petitioned to remain in the UK on compassionate grounds due to the life-threatening nature of her illness and lack of accessible treatment in her home country.

In the heated public debate about Sumani's case, some British physicians and other sympathetic observers argued that her forcible removal constituted a gross human rights violation. A *Lancet* editorial labeled it an act of "atrocious barbarism" and anticipated that her deportation would precipitate her death (*Lancet* 2008). Yet several Members of Parliament vocally supported the Home Office actions. Without denying the likelihood of her imminent death, they claimed her case failed to meet the necessary threshold of "very exceptional" suffering required to activate the country's humanitarian relief mechanism.

Ultimately, the judge reviewing Sumani's case deemed her situation unexceptional, and her appeal was denied (Lawrance 2012). Five British Home Office agents moved her into a wheelchair, drove her to Heathrow Airport, and put her on a plane to Ghana against her will. Unable to access treatment in her country of origin, she died two months later.

The geographic and temporal contexts in which Sumani's case was decided are crucial to understanding the way her deservingness was reckoned. In the UK, healthcare provision to migrant populations historically has been uncontroversial, and until relatively recently access to care was virtually the same for all. After an increase in asylum applications in the 1970s and 1980s, however, anxieties about growing migrant populations spurred the passage of laws distinguishing between "ordinary residents" eligible for free healthcare through the National Health Service and "non-ordinary residents" who can access only certain health services, and only for a fee (*Lancet* 2008). Sumani's January 2008 removal from the UK also took place at a crucial point in global economic history—the onset of the Great Recession. Though she would not live long enough to know it, the economic downturn between 2007 and 2009 would ultimately precipitate a decade of austerity measures in the UK, including substantial cuts to health care among other forms of public spending. In an earlier time, Sumani might have received greater humanitarian consideration. Were she alive in post-Brexit UK, she might have had even greater difficulty obtaining appropriate care as an "undesirable" African immigrant.

Sumani might also have fared differently if she had lived just across the English Channel, in France. In both the UK and France, African migrants face discrimination. At the time of Sumani's removal, however, French policies regarding sick migrants tended to be more favorable than their British analogs. In 1998, following an intensive campaign by a coalition of advocacy organizations, an informal, discretionary practice of granting temporary residency permits to seriously ill migrants became institutionalized (Ticktin 2011; Fassin 2012). The resulting new arrangement, an "illness residency permit," was created precisely to prevent the deportation of people with serious illnesses who would lack access to appropriate care following repatriation—people like Ama Sumani.

On the surface, the contours of the French and UK policies are similar. Both revolve around the same questions: Does the migrant's illness meet the threshold of "life-threatening" severity? Would appropriate treatment be accessible in his or her home country? What differs is the deservingness threshold, which would appear to be lower in France. Importantly, medical experts play an integral role in the French context, whereas immigration officers are the primary adjudicators in the UK (Fassin 2012; Larchanché 2012; Ticktin 2011).

Might Sumani still be alive had she migrated to France instead of the UK? We can never know. But her case serves as an important, if tragic, illustration of how consequential context can be to constructions of health-related deservingness, and in turn, how health-related deservingness narratives can become matters of life and death.

"Pirate" Daycares and Infant Deaths in Israel

During a six-week period in early 2015, five infants died in Tel Aviv, Israel, in what advocates and the media described as "pirate" daycares, or "child warehouses," in the city's neglected southern neighborhoods.[5] Among them were two four-month-old babies who died within a forty-eight-hour period. The local media were quick to publicize these deaths (see, for example, David 2015; Kashti 2015; Vilnai 2015a, 2015b, 2015c), both involving infants born in Israel to Eritrean parents who had arrived, without authorization, seeking asylum.

In the first of these cases, a baby girl was left alone in a crib with a bottle of formula (Vilnai 2015b), possibly tied to her head (David 2015), and choked to death. The next day, in an adjacent neighborhood, a baby boy died of suffocation; his death went unnoticed until his mother came to pick him up after work and found him lying on his stomach, unresponsive. Immediately after this pair of deaths, migrant advocacy organizations and human rights groups demanded swift government action, and the media reported on "marathon meetings" in the subsequent days "among the relevant government ministries, in collaboration with the municipality"

(Vilnai 2015c). Had the deceased infants been born to Jewish-Israeli citizen parents rather than non-Jewish asylum seekers from Africa, how might their fates have been different?

For nearly two decades, "pirate" daycares like these have been the only viable option for most infants and toddlers (age 0–3) born in Israel to unauthorized migrant parents, including both migrants who arrived explicitly in search of work and those, like the Eritrean parents of these unfortunate children, who arrived seeking asylum. Although asylum-seekers in Israel are officially forbidden to work, they receive no benefits from the government and therefore must find employment in order to sustain themselves and their families. Their employment options are thus sharply limited, pay is low, work conditions are often harsh, and parents have little flexibility in determining their work schedules. As a result, some children are in daycare for fifteen hours per day or more—or even overnight, in some cases for multiple nights in succession.

Significantly, no public daycare frameworks are provided for any children in this age bracket, including Israeli citizens' children. Yet the private daycares that serve Israeli parents face tighter scrutiny—not only from the authorities, but also from parents who, as citizens, risk little in voicing their concerns.

As of 2015, an estimated seventy to eighty "pirate" daycares were operating in the Tel Aviv area, serving approximately 2,500 children and charging as little as 500 Israeli shekels (approximately US$132) per month for care that often exceeds what counts as "full-time" by Israeli standards (Vilnai 2015b; Mesila staff, personal interview). For Israeli politicians, the media, and the broader public, this spate of deaths came as no surprise; in the preceding two years, at least ten others had been recorded in similar settings (Vilnai 2015c). Indeed, the risks and dangers of these unregulated daycares had been detailed and roundly condemned in the State Comptroller's 2013 annual report (Office of the State Comptroller 2013).

Thousands of children do survive these settings, but the short- and long-term risks are legion—and well-known. In many such daycares, a single adult, usually a woman with a migrant background, is responsible for as many as twenty or even thirty children (Office of the State Comptroller 2013) whereas the national average ratio in Israel is one to six (David 2015). As a result, children tend to spend as many as twelve to fifteen hours each day isolated in a crib with no daily routine and with minimal attention, physical contact, or direct interaction with others, whether children or adults. Neither do they receive much stimulation (e.g., stories, toys, music, art activities, outdoor playtime), although televisions are sometimes present. Most facilities are located in crumbling residential buildings, often in private apartments where rents are cheap. Among other hazards, many lack fire escapes and adequate ventilation, and some have unauthorized electrical connections, unsecured doors or gates, and unsafe balconies.

From a health standpoint, the long-term impact of spending one's critical first years in a setting like this is almost universally devastating. According to Mesila, a municipally run social welfare organization in South Tel Aviv that had been responding to these unregulated care settings and their effects for more than a decade: "By the time they enter formal educational settings, every one of these children suffers at least one if not more forms of developmental delay" (Mesila Aid and Information Center 2006). They continue: "we are convinced that the overwhelming majority of infants and young children in these frameworks meet the criteria for children at risk as a result of spending most hours of the day in an atmosphere of physical and emotional deprivation that severely delays their development" (Mesila Aid and Information Center 2006). These conclusions were echoed in the 2013 State Comptroller report.

What "common-sense" assumptions and moral commitments make it possible for key stakeholders in the political and policy realms to ignore these well-known risks for years, even decades? The infants who died certainly could not be suspected of poor moral character. In terms of migration motive, they were neither economic nor forced migrants; although their parents fled countries in tumult, they were born in Israel. Since Israel has no *jus soli* provision, however, they are not eligible for Israeli citizenship.

One might expect that their young age and associated vulnerability would garner concern for their health and development, and in some respects, this has been the case. Since the 2000s, children of migrant parents have been among the few members of migrant communities for whom national and municipal stakeholders have expressed concern. For example, a small network of supervised private daycares (Unitaf) was established under the supervision of Mesila in 2005, with major philanthropic (as opposed to government) support. Unitaf daycares are roughly comparable to those serving Jewish-Israeli children, but they are more expensive for parents than the informal arrangements described above—and they have too few places to meet local demand.

Changes benefiting these children have been driven both by pressure from local migrant and child advocacy groups and, not insignificantly, by a cultural emphasis on children and reproduction that has long found expression in the country's robust and institutionalized tradition of (selective) pronatalism (Kahn 2000; Kanaaneh 2002). Yet the overriding factor shaping Israeli attitudes toward children of migrant parents is social proximity. The clearest illustration of how proximity is reckoned in Israel is the country's "Law of Return." Established to invert the genocidal logic of the Nazi regime, this legal provision offers full citizenship benefits to anyone with a bureaucratically legible tie to the Jewish people. For those who lack such a tie, however, citizenship, and even permanent resident status, are almost completely unattainable regardless of country of origin or current legal status.

On the basis of this ethnonational logic, virtually everyone residing in Israel falls into one of three groups: ratified citizens (Jewish-Israelis, including the native-born and immigrants arriving under the Law of Return); Palestinians (who are represented as the country's "real" Others); and "other" Others—global migrants who have arrived in Israel for a variety of economic and/or political reasons and cannot readily be slotted into either of the first two groups (Willen 2019). For the vast majority of politicians, policymakers, and citizens, societal attention, investment, and care ought to focus primarily—some would say exclusively—on the country's Jewish-Israeli citizens. Other groups are constructed not simply as undeserving, but as a threat to the country's economy, identity, and even in some instances its existential security.

Immediately after this wave of infant deaths, the Prime Minister's Office announced it would begin working with Mesila to scale-up the small network of Unitaf daycares (which would continue to rely heavily on support from private philanthropy) (Mesila Aid and Information Center 2015). It is impossible to know precisely how key stakeholders' responses might have differed had the deceased infants been born to Jewish-Israeli citizen parents rather than African asylum seekers. Given the contours of Israel's "local moral economy" (Willen 2019), however, it seems likely that state, local, and non-government actors, under pressure from citizens and the media, would have responded much sooner—and with considerably greater decisiveness.

Conclusion

In this chapter, we have argued that social scientists' capacity to understand—and intervene in—debates about migration, and especially about migrants' health, depends on our ability to understand how deservingness is reckoned by local actors espousing divergent values, commitments, and agendas. To this end, we presented an analytical framework that highlights the key role of stakeholders, contextual factors, and evaluative criteria in debates about health-related deservingness. As the deservingness debates analyzed here make clear, conceptions of deservingness are fundamentally expressed in a moral register; they are vernacular expressions of value as opposed to juridical notions of right. As such, deservingness inevitably is reckoned in ways that are relational, conditional, context-dependent, syncretic, affect-laden, and mutable. Put simply, deservingness assessments are rooted in moral, ideological, and political assumptions that reflect different—and competing—forms of "common sense."

Of course, common sense reflects hegemonic narratives and understandings of past and present; of inclusion and exclusion; and above all of what, and who, matters. In the present era, we are seeing the emergence—or, perhaps more accurately, the resurgence—of divergent modes of common sense and deeply conflicting systems of cultural hegemony (Gramsci 1971). Factors contributing to these cleavages, many of them driven by technological "advances," include intensive media polarization; the erosion of confidence in once-broadly credible institutions and sources of authority (e.g., journalists, scientists, political leaders); and the diminishing role of empirical evidence in public and policy debates—itself a matter of grave and urgent concern. The possibility of lightning-fast digital communication and the widespread use (including overuse) of social media play central roles as well. These are the circumstances that make it possible, for example, for a Trump administration official to radically reinterpret Emma Lazarus's poem on the fly, during a nationally broadcast radio interview, to insist that migrants are welcome in the United States only if they "can stand on their own two feet and . . . will not become a public charge."

In closing, we highlight two areas of inquiry that demand further attention. First, we know altogether too little about how different groups of migrants—and members of other vulnerable groups—conceptualize their own deservingness. What sort of social contracts do they perceive, envision, or hope for? How do they participate in, or respond to, the frequently contentious deservingness debates transpiring in their communities of residence (and, at times, swirling around them)? What barriers impede their ability to speak out and participate in these debates on their own behalf? These questions all demand closer scrutiny.

Second, it is increasingly evident that racism, discrimination, and other forms of oppression and exclusion impair health and shorten lives (see, e.g., Bailey et al 2017; Castañeda 2019; Castañeda et al. 2015; Holmes 2013; Horton 2016). The violent effects of racism have emerged with chilling clarity as racialized individuals and communities have faced dramatically heightened rates of COVID-19 infection, and mortality, relative to those racialized as white (Bowleg 2020; Devakumar et al. 2020; Gee et al. 2020; Hardeman et al. 2020). What are the health effects for migrants and their families of being made to feel unwelcome and undeserving of society's attention, investment, or care? We need to engage such questions with robust epidemiological methods and evidence (Orcutt et al. 2020), but that is but one vital step. By listening to migrants, foregrounding their experience, and supporting their efforts to speak publicly on their own behalf, anthropologists can contribute in vital ways to conversations—in the academy and beyond—about how exclusion and sociopolitical abjection harm health, and we can support migrants' efforts to lead dignified and flourishing lives (Willen et al., 2021).

Only with strong tools and robust conceptual frameworks can we begin to parse the messy and confusing reality of the early twenty-first century—an era in which notions of the collective "we" are proving more fragile than many of us would have hoped, and in which some would exile even Lady Liberty, that silent-lipped "Mother of Exiles," from the American body politic.

Acknowledgments

An earlier version of this chapter was published in Thomas, Felicia, ed. 2016. *The Handbook of Migration and Health*. Cheltenham, UK: Edward Elgar. Portions of the chapter draw on "How Is Health-Related "Deservingness" Reckoned?" and the introduction to a Social Science and Medicine special issue titled, "Migration, 'Illegality', and Health: Mapping Embodied Vulnerability and Debating Health-Related Deservingness" by Sarah S. Willen.

Sarah S. Willen is Associate Professor of Anthropology at the University of Connecticut and Director of the Research Program on Global Health & Human Rights at UConn's Human Rights Institute. She has written widely on a range of topics, including the phenomenology of illegalization, migration and health, health-related deservingness, and the lived pursuits of dignity and flourishing. Willen's books include the multiple award winning *Fighting for Dignity: Migrant Lives at Israel's Margins* (University of Pennsylvania Press, 2019). She is also Principal Investigator of ARCHES | the AmeRicans' Conceptions of Health Equity Study and Co-Founder of the Pandemic Journaling Project.

Jennifer Cook is a Research Associate with the Tower Center for International Affairs and Public Policy at Southern Methodist University. After receiving her PhD in Anthropology from the University of Connecticut in May 2017, she completed a three-year Postdoctoral Fellowship with the Tower Center (2017–2020). Cook's research program focuses on Mexico-United States migration, transnational family and labor issues, and im/migrant il/legality. Her current book project, tentatively titled *Lawful Permanent Migrant: Legality and Mobility in Transnational Mexico*, uses multi-sited ethnographic methods to examine the way legal immigrant status transforms life in transnational Mexican communities.

Notes

1. "Morning Edition." *NPR*, 13 August 2019. https://www.npr.org/2019/08/13/750727515/rule-would-penalize-immigrants-to-u-s-for-needing-benefits.
2. Although the terms "migrant" and "immigrant" often are used interchangeably, they are not synonymous. Often these terms are employed as ostensibly neutral, empirically grounded descriptors of particular individuals or groups, yet different terms convey different ideological messages about who is expected to keep moving and who deserves to stay. Since individuals on the move often do not—and perhaps cannot—know whether their residence in a given location is temporary or permanent, or what sort of status will ultimately be available to them, the open-ended terms "migrants" and "migration" hew closest to the variability, as well as the uncertainty, associated with many contemporary patterns of human mobility.
3. Sumani arrived in the UK in 2003 on a tourist visa. She later obtained a student visa and enrolled in finance classes, but her poor English skills and insufficient educational preparation prevented her from completing her course of study. Her myeloma was diagnosed in 2006, and she was placed on dialysis after the cancer spread to her kidneys. The Home Office ordered her "removal" to Ghana, arguing that her employment violated the terms of her student visa (Lawrance 2012).
4. In the UK, the response to visa violations is "removal," which does not affect a migrant's opportunity to apply for future visas, rather than "deportation," which does. Migrants may be deported if they have committed crimes or entered illegally (Blinder 2015).
5. Data for this section draw on ethnographic research conducted by the first author in Tel Aviv in 2014, supplemented by official reports and media coverage. This research phase, part of a larger study initiated in 2000, included interviews with staff at Mesila; visits to three "pirate" daycares; and an interview with the head of a Unitaf daycare.

References

Appelbaum, Lauren D. 2001. "The Influence of Perceived Deservingness on Policy Decisions Regarding Aid to the Poor." *Political Psychology* 22(3): 419–42.

Appelbaum, Lauren D., Mary Clare Lennon, and John Lawrence Aber. 2003. "How Belief in a Just World Influences Views of Public Policy." *National Center for Children in Poverty, Columbia University*. Retrieved 7 February from www.nccp.org/publications/pub_553.html.

Bailey, Zinzi D., Nancy Krieger, Madina Agénor, Jasmine Graves, Natalia Linos, and Mary T. Bassett. 2017. "Structural Racism and Health Inequities in the USA: Evidence and Interventions." *The Lancet* 389(10077): 1453–63.

Bambra, Clare, and Katherine E. Smith. 2010. "No Longer Deserving? Sickness Benefit Reform and the Politics of (Ill) Health." *Critical Public Health* 20(1): 71–84.

Blekesaune, Morten, and Jill Quadagno. 2003. "Public Attitudes toward Welfare State Policies." *European Sociological Review* 19(5): 415–27.

Blinder, Scott. 2015. *Briefing: Deportations, Removals, and Voluntary Departures from the UK*, 3rd revision, Oxford, Migration Observatory at the University of Oxford. .

Blomberg, Helena, Johanna Kallio, Olli Kangas, Christian Kroll, and Mikko Niemelä . 2017. "Social Assistance Deservingness and Policy Measures: Attitudes of Finnish Politicians, Administrators and Citizens." *In* Wim van Oorschot, Femke Roosma, Bart Meuleman, Tim Reeskens (Eds.), 2017. *The Social Legitimacy of Targeted Welfare: Attitudes to Welfare Deservingness*. Edward Elgar: Cheltenham, UK. pp. 209–24.

Bourgois, Philippe, Seth M. Holmes, Kim Sue, and James Quesada. 2017. "Structural Vulnerability: Operationalizing the Concept to Address Health Disparities in Clinical Care." *Academic Medicine* 92(3): 299–307.

Bowleg, Lisa. 2020. "We're Not All in This Together: On COVID-19, Intersectionality, and Structural Inequality." *American Journal of Public Health* 110(7): 917.

Carruth, Lauren Carlos Martinez, Lahra Smith, Katharine Donato, Carlos Piñones-Rivera, and James Quesada. 2021. "Structural Vulnerability: Migration, Healthcare, and Structures that Make Us All Vulnerable." *BMJ-Global Health* 6(Supplement 1): e005109.

Castañeda, Heide. 2019. *Borders of Belonging: Struggle and Solidarity in Mixed-Status Immigrant Families*. Stanford, CA: Stanford University Press.

Castañeda, Heide, Seth M. Holmes, Daniel S. Madrigal, Maria-Elena DeTrinidad Young, Naomi Beyeler, and James Quesada. 2015. "Immigration as a Social Determinant of Health." *Annual Review of Public Health* 36: 375–92.

Chauvin, Sébastien, and Blanca Garcés-Mascareñas. 2014. "Becoming Less Illegal: Deservingness Frames and Undocumented Migrant Incorporation." *Sociology Compass* 8(4): 422–32.

Chauvin, Sébastien, Blanca Garcés-Mascareñas, and Albert Kraler. 2013. "Employment and Migrant Deservingness." *International Migration* 51(6): 80–85.

Chavez, Leo R. 2006. "Imagining the Nation, Imagining Donor Recipients." In *A Death Retold*, ed. Keith Wailoo, Julie Livingston, and Peter Guarnaccia. Chapel Hill: University of North Carolina Press.

———. 2012. "Undocumented Immigrants and Their Use of Medical Services in Orange County, California." *Social Science and Medicine* 74(6): 887–93.

Chock, Phyllis Pease. 1991. "'Illegal Aliens' and 'Opportunity': Myth-Making in Congressional Testimony." *American Ethnologist* 18(2): 279–94.

Council of Europe. 1950. *European Convention for the Protection of Human Rights and Fundamental Freedoms, as amended by Protocols Nos. 11 and 14*, ETS 5. Retrieved 7 February 2022 from www.refworld.org/docid/3ae6b3b04.html.

Daniels, Norman. 2008. *Just Health*. Cambridge: Cambridge University Press.

David, Ariel. 2015. "Who Will Save the Refugee Children of Tel Aviv?" *Ha'aretz*, 5 April. Retrieved 7 February 2022 from www.haaretz.com/news/israel/.premium-1.650425.

de Swaan, Abram. 1988. *In Care of the State*. New York: Oxford University Press.

de Vries, Robert. 2017. "Negative Attitudes towards Welfare Claimants: The Importance of Unconscious Bias. Claimants." In *The Social Legitimacy of Targeted Welfare: Attitudes to Welfare Deservingness*, eds. Wim van Oorschot, Femke Roosma, Bart Meuleman, Tim Reeskens. Edward Elgar: Cheltenham, UK. pp. 93–112.

de Wilde, Marjolijn. 2017. "Deservingness in Social Assistance Administrative Practice: A Factorial Survey Approach." In *The Social Legitimacy of Targeted Welfare: Attitudes to Welfare Deservingness*, eds. Wim van Oorschot, Femke Roosma, Bart Meuleman, Tim Reeskens. Edward Elgar: Cheltenham, UK. Pp. 225–40.

Devakumar, Delan, Sujitha Selvarajah, Geordan Shannon, Kui Muraya, Sarah Lasoye, Susanna Corona, Yin Paradies, Ibrahim Abubakar, and E. Tendayi Achiume. 2020. "Racism, the Public Health Crisis We Can No Longer Ignore." *The Lancet* 395(10242): e112–e113.

el-Shaarawi, Nadia. 2021. "A Transit State: The Ambivalences of the Refugee Resettlement Process for Iraqis in Cairo." *American Ethnologist* 48(4: 404–17.

Fassin, Didier. 2012. *Humanitarian Reason*. Berkeley: University of California Press.

Feather, Norman T. 1999. *Values, Achievement, and Justice*. New York: Kluwer Academic/Plenum.

Gee, Gilbert C., Marguerite J. Ro, and Anne W. Rimoin. 2020. "Seven reasons to care about racism and COVID-19 and seven things to do to stop it." *American Journal of Public Health* 110(7): 954–55.

Geiger, Ben Baumberg. 2017. "False Beliefs and the Perceived Deservingness of Social Security Benefit Claimants." In *The Social Legitimacy of Targeted Welfare: Attitudes to Welfare Deservingness*, eds. Wim van Oorschot, Femke Roosma, Bart Meuleman, Tim Reeskens. Edward Elgar: Cheltenham, UK. pp. 73–92.

Gilens, Martin. 1999. *Why Americans Hate Welfare*. Chicago: University of Chicago Press.

Gollust, Sarah E., Paula M. Lantz, and Peter A. Ubel. 2010. "The Polarizing Effect of News Media Messages about the Social Determinants of Health." *American Journal of Public Health* 99(12): 2160–67.

Gollust, Sarah E., and Julia Lynch. 2010. *Who Deserves Health Care?* Robert Wood Johnson Foundation Working Paper Series (WP-48).

Gottlieb, Nora, Dani Filc, and Nadav Davidovitch. 2012. "Medical Humanitarianism, Human Rights, and Political Advocacy." *Social Science and Medicine* 74(6): 839–45.

Gramsci, Antonio. 1971. *Selections from the Prison Notebooks*, edited and translated by Quintin Hoare and Geoffrey Nowell Smith. London: Lawrence & Wishar.

Grove, Natalie J., and Anthony B. Zwi. 2006. "Our Health and Theirs: Forced Migration, Othering, and Public Health." *Social Science and Medicine* 62(8): 1931–42.

Guetzkow, Joshua. 2010. "Beyond Deservingness: Congressional Discourse on Poverty, 1964–1996." *Annals of the American Academy of Political and Social Science* 629(1): 173–97.

Haas, Bridget M. 2017. "Citizens-in-Waiting, Deportees-in-Waiting: Power, Temporality, and Suffering in the U.S. Asylum System." *Ethos* 45(1): 75-97.

Hardeman, Rachel R., Eduardo M. Medina and Rhea W. Boyd. 2020. "Stolen Breaths." *New England Journal of Medicine* 383(3): 197–99.

Heyman, Josian. 1998. *Finding a Moral Heart for US Immigration Policy*. Washington, DC: American Anthropological Association.

Holmes, Seth M. 2012. "The Clinical Gaze in the Practice of Migrant Health." *Social Science and Medicine* 74(6): 873–81.

———. 2013. *Fresh Fruit, Broken Bodies*. Oakland: University of California Press.

Holmes, Seth M., Ernesto Castañeda, Jeremy Geeraert, Heide Castañeda, Ursula Probst, Nina Zeldes, Sarah S. Willen, Yusupha Dibba, Raphael Frankfurter, Anne Kveim Lie, John Fredrik Askjer, Heidi Fjeld. 2021. "Deservingness: migration and health in social context." *BMJ Global Health* 6(Suppl 1): e005107.

Horton, Sarah. 2004. "Different Subjects: The Health Care System's Participation in the Differential Construction of the Cultural Citizenship of Cuban Refugees and Mexican Immigrants." *Medical Anthropology Quarterly* 18(4): 472–89.

———. 2016. *They Leave Their Kidneys in the Field.* Oakland: University of California Press.

Huschke, Susann. 2014. "Performing Deservingness: Humanitarian Health Care Provision for Migrants in Germany." *Social Science and Medicine* 120: 352–59.

Kahn, Susan. 2000. *Reproducing Jews.* Durham, NC: Duke University Press.

Kanaaneh, Rhoda Ann. 2002. *Birthing the Nation.* Berkeley: University of California Press.

Kashti, Or. 2015. "Israeli Government's Apathy is Killing Foreign Workers' Children." *Ha'aretz* newspaper, 31 March. Retrieved 7 February 2022 from www.haaretz.com/opinion/.premium-1.649736.

Katz, Michael B. 1989. *The Undeserving Poor.* New York: Pantheon Books.Kline, Nolan. 2019. "When Deservingness Policies Converge: US Immigration Enforcement, Health Reform and Patient Dumping." *Anthropology & Medicine* 26(3): 280–95.

Kochhar, Rakesh, Roberto Ruro, and Sonya Tafoya. 2005. *The New Latino South.* Washington, DC: Pew Hispanic Center.

Kootstra, Anouk. 2016. "Deserving and Undeserving Welfare Claimants in Britain and the Netherlands: Examining the Role of Ethnicity and Migration Status Using a Vignette Experiment." *European Sociological Review* 32(3): 325–38.

Kovacs, Joe. 2003. "Transplants for Illegals Igniting US Firestorm." *World Net Daily*, 6 March. Retrieved 7 February 2022 from www.wnd.com/2003/03/17606.

Lancet. 2008. "Migrant Health: What Are Doctors' Leaders Doing?" *Lancet* 371(9608): P178.

Larchanché, Stéphanie. 2012. "Intangible Obstacles: Health Implications of Stigmatization, Structural Violence, and Fear among Undocumented Immigrants in France." *Social Science and Medicine* 74(6): 858–63.

———. 2020. *Cultural Anxieties: Managing Migrant Suffering in France.* New Brunswick, NJ: Rutgers University Press.

Lawrance, Benjamin N. 2012. "Humanitarian Claims and Expert Testimonies." *Ghana Studies* 15/16: 251–86.

Lepianka, Dorota. 2017. "The Varying Faces of Poverty and Deservingness in Dutch Print Media." In *The Social Legitimacy of Targeted Welfare: Attitudes to Welfare Deservingness*, eds. Wim van Oorschot, Femke Roosma, Bart Meuleman, Tim Reeskens. Edward Elgar: Cheltenham, UK. pp. 127–48.

Lipsky, Michael. 1980. *Street-Level Bureaucracy.* New York: Russell Sage Foundation.

Lynch, Julia, and Sarah E. Gollust. 2010. *Playing Fair: Fairness Beliefs and Health Policy Preferences in the United States.* Robert Wood Johnson Foundation Working Paper Series (WP-47).

Malkin, Michelle. 2003. "America: Medical Welcome Mat to the World." *VDare*, 20 February. Retrieved 7 February 2022 from www.vdare.com/articles/america-medical-welcome-mat-to-the-world.Maness, Sarah B., Laura Merrell, Erika L. Thompson, Stacey B. Griner, Nolan Kline, and Christopher Wheldon. 2020. "Social Determinants of Health and Health Disparities: COVID-19 Exposures and Mortality among African American People in the United States." *Public Health Reports* 136(1):18–22.

Marrow, Helen. 2011. "Deserving to a Point: Undocumented Immigrants in San Francisco's Universal Access Healthcare Model." *Social Science and Medicine* 74(6): 846–54.

Marrow, Helen, and Tiffany D. Joseph. 2015. "Excluded and Frozen Out: Unauthorized Immigrants' (Non)access to Care after US Health Care Reform." *Journal of Ethnic and Migration Studies* 41(14): 2253–73.

Mesila Aid and Information Center. 2006. *Annual Activity Report.* Tel Aviv: Mesila Aid and Information Center.

———. 2015. *Summer 2015 at Mesila.* Tel Aviv: Mesila Aid and Information Center.

Morgen, Sandra, and Jeff Maskovsky. 2003. "The Anthropology of Welfare 'Reform.'" *Annual Review of Anthropology* 32: 315–38.

Newton, Lina. 2005. "It Is Not a Question of Being Anti-Immigration." In *Deserving and Entitled,* ed. Anne Schneider and Helen Ingram, 139–72. Albany, NY: SUNY Press.

Ngai, Mae M. 2004. *Impossible Subjects.* Princeton, NJ: Princeton University Press.

Office of the State Comptroller. 2013. *Annual Report.* Retrieved 7 February 2022 from https://www.mevaker.gov.il/sites/DigitalLibrary/Pages/Reports/244-48.aspx.

Oliverio-Lauderdale, Daniela. 2014. "Contradictions and Exclusions: An Ethnographic Study of African Im/migrants' Right to Health in Italy." MA Thesis. Vancouver: University of British Columbia.

Olsen, Jan Abel, Jeff Richardson, Paul Dolan, and Paul Menzel. 2003. "The Moral Relevance of Personal Characteristics in Setting Health Care Priorities." *Social Science and Medicine* 57(7): 1163–72.Orcutt, Miriam, Parth Patel, Rachel Burns, Lucinda Hiam, Rob Aldridge, Delan Devakumar, Bernadette Kumar, Paul Spiegel, and Ibrahim Abubakar. 2020. "Global Call to Action for Inclusion of Migrants and Refugees in the COVID-19 Response." *The Lancet* 395: 1482–83.

Portes, Alejandro, Patricia Fernández-Kelly, and Donald Light. 2012. "Life on the Edge: Immigrants Confront the American Health System." *Ethnic and Racial Studies* 35(1): 3–22.

Quesada, James, Laurie Kain Hart, and Philippe Bourgois. 2011. "Structural Vulnerability and Health." *Medical Anthropology* 30(4): 339–62.

Ragusa, Jordan. 2017. "Do the Rich Deserve a Tax Cut? Public Images, Deservingness Criteria and Americans' Tax Policy Preferences." In *The Social Legitimacy of Targeted Welfare: Attitudes to Welfare Deservingness,* eds. Wim van Oorschot, Femke Roosma, Bart Meuleman, Tim Reeskens. Edward Elgar: Cheltenham, UK. pp. 316–34.

Roosma, Femke and Marjolein Jeene. 2017. "The Deservingness Logic Applied to Public Opinions Concerning Work Obligatinos for Benefits Claimants." In *The Social Legitimacy of Targeted Welfare: Attitudes to Welfare Deservingness,* eds. Wim van Oorschot, Femke Roosma, Bart Meuleman, Tim Reeskens. Edward Elgar: Cheltenham, UK. pp. 189–08.

Rylko-Bauer, Barbara, and Paul Farmer. 2002. "Managed Care or Managed Inequality? A Call for Critiques of Market-Based Medicine." *Medical Anthropology Quarterly* 16(4): 476–502.

Sadin, Meredith. 2017. "They're Not Worthy: The Perceived Deservingness of the Rich and its Connection to Policy Preferences." In *The Social Legitimacy of Targeted Welfare: Attitudes to Welfare Deservingness,* eds. Wim van Oorschot, Femke Roosma, Bart Meuleman, Tim Reeskens. Edward Elgar: Cheltenham, UK. pp. 299–15.

Sales, Rosemary. 2002. "The Deserving and the Undeserving? Refugees, Asylum Seekers and Welfare in Britain." *Critical Social Policy* 22(3): 456–78.

Schneider, Anne L., and Helen M. Ingram. 2005. *Deserving and Entitled: Social Constructions and Public Policy.* Albany, NY: SUNY Press.

Scott, Charity. 2008. "Belief in a Just World." *Hastings Center Report* 38(1): 16–19.

Streinzer, Andreas, and Jelena Tošić. Forthcoming. "Introduction: Deservingness: Reassessing the Moral Dimensions of Inequality." In *Ethnographies of Deservingness: Unpacking Ideologies of Distribution and Inequality,* ed. Andreas Streinzer and Jelena Tošić. New York: Berghahn Books.

Stumpf, Juliet P. 2006. "The Crimmigration Crisis." *American University Law Review* 56: 367–418.

Snell-Rood, Claire, and Elizabeth Carpenter-Song. 2018. "Depression in a Depressed Area: Deservingness, Mental Illness, and Treatment in the Contemporary Rural US." *Social Science and Medicine* 219: 78–86.

Ticktin, Miriam. 2011. *Casualties of Care*. Berkeley: University of California Press.

Tiedje, Kristina, and David J. Plevak. 2014. "Medical Humanitarianism in the United States: Alternative Healthcare, Spirituality, and Political Advocacy in the Case of Our Lady Guadalupe Free Clinic." *Social Science and Medicine* 120: 360–67.

Tošić, Jelena, and Andreas Streinzer, eds. Forthcoming. *Ethnographies of Deservingness: Unpacking Ideologies of Distribution and Inequality*. New York: Berghahn Books.

Van Doorn, Bas and Angela Bos. 2017. "Are Visual Depictions of Poverty in the US Gendered and Racialized?" In *The Social Legitimacy of Targeted Welfare: Attitudes to Welfare Deservingness*, eds. Wim van Oorschot, Femke Roosma, Bart Meuleman, Tim Reeskens. Edward Elgar: Cheltenham, UK. pp. 113–26.

van Oorschot, Wim. 2000. "Who Should Get What, and Why? On Deservingness Criteria and the Conditionality of Solidarity among the Public." *Policy & Politics* 28(1): 33–48.

———. 2006. "Making the Difference in Social Europe." *Journal of European Social Policy*, 16(1): 23–42.

van Oorschot, Wim, Femke Roosma, Bart Meuleman, and Tim Reeskens, eds. 2017. *The Social Legitimacy of Targeted Welfare: Attitudes to Welfare Deservingness*. Cheltenham, Glos, UK: Edward Elgar.

Vanthuyne, Karine, Francesca Meloni, Monica Ruiz-Casares, Cécile Rousseau, and Alexandra Ricard-Guay. 2013. "Health Workers' Perceptions of Access to Care for Children and Pregnant Women with Precarious Immigration Status." *Social Science & Medicine* 93: 78–85.

Verkuyten, Maykel. 2004. "Emotional Reactions to and Support for Immigrant Policies." *Social Justice Research* 17(3): 293–314.

Viladrich, Anahi. 2012. "Beyond Welfare Reform: Reframing Undocumented Immigrants' Entitlement to Health Care in the United States." *Social Science and Medicine* 74(6): 822–29.

———. 2019. "'We Cannot Let Them Die': Undocumented Immigrants and Media Framing of Health Deservingness in the United States." *Qualitative Health Research* 29(10): 1447–60.

Vilnai, Orly. 2015a. "Three Infants Died this Month Because of Harsh Conditions on Daycares for Children of Asylum Seekers." *Ha'aretz*, 25 February. Retrieved 7 February 2022 from www.haaretz.co.il/news/orly/.premium-1.2573759.

———. 2015b. "Four-Month-Old Infant Dies in Daycare for Children of Asylum Seekers in South Tel Aviv." *Ha'aretz*, 29 March. Retrieved 7 February 2022 from www.haaretz.co.il/news/education/.premium-1.2601973.

———. 2015c. "Another Infant Dies in the 'Child Warehouses' in South Tel Aviv, the Fifth in Two Months." *Ha'aretz*, 30 March. Retrieved 7 February 2022 from www.haaretz.co.il/news/education/1.2602929.

Wailoo, Keith, Julie Livingston, and Peter Guarnaccia, eds. 2006. *A Death Retold: Jesica Santillan, the Bungled Transplant, and Paradoxes of Medical Citizenship*. Chapel Hill: University of North Carolina Press.

Watters, Charles. 2007. "Refugees at Europe's Borders: The Moral Economy of Care." *Transcultural Psychiatry* 44(3): 394–417.

Will, Jeffry A. 1993. "The Dimensions of Poverty: Public Perceptions of the Deserving Poor." *Social Science Research* 22(3): 312–32.

Willen, Sarah S. 2011. "Do 'Illegal' Migrants Have a 'Right to Health'? Engaging Ethical Theory as Social Practice at a Tel Aviv Open Clinic." *Medical Anthropology Quarterly* 45(3): 303–30.

———. 2012a. "How is Health-Related 'Deservingness' Reckoned?" *Social Science and Medicine* 74(6): 812–21.

———, ed. 2012b. "Special Issue—Migration, 'Illegality', and Health: Mapping Embodied Vulnerability and Debating Health-related Deservingness." *Social Science and Medicine* 74(6): 805–11.

———. 2019. *Fighting for Dignity: Migrant Lives at Israel's Margins*. Philadelphia: University of Pennsylvania Press.

Willen, Sarah S., Nasima Selim, Emily Mendenhall, Miriam Magaña Lopez, Shahanoor Chowdhury, and Hansjörg Dilger. 2021. "Flourishing: Migration and Health in Social Context." *BMJ-Global Health*. 6(Suppl 1): e005108.

WHO Commission on Social Determinants of Health. 2008. *Closing the Gap in a Generation: Health Equity through Action on the Social Determinants of Health*. Geneva: World Health Organization.

Yarris, Kristin, and Heide Castañeda, eds. 2015. "Special Issue—Discourses of Displacement and Deservingness: Interrogating Distinctions between 'Economic' and 'Forced' Migration." *International Migration* 53(3): 64–69.

Yoo, Grace J. 2002. "Constructing Deservingness." *Journal of Aging and Social Policy* 13: 17–34.

———. 2008. "Immigrants and Welfare: Policy Constructions of Deservingness." *Journal of Immigrant and Refugee Studies* 6(4): 490–507.

2

Wanting to "Be Seen"

Experiences of Migration, Gender, and Motherhood in Johannesburg, South Africa

Rebecca Walker and Elsa Oliveira

Cities all over the world defy easy characterization. They can be simultaneously vibrant and chaotic, spaces of high visibility and invisibility, places of opportunity and, at the same time, marginalization. While cities are often where people go in search of improved livelihoods, cities can also be where some of the most extreme human rights violations occur.

Often referred to as the "City of Gold"—Johannesburg (one of South Africa's three main cities) is a place where many South Africans and foreign-born nationals come in search of better lives. Yet few of its residents call the city home (Landau 2006). For some, Johannesburg represents a place of hope, refuge and creativity whereas for others, it is a place of abject poverty, violence, and decay. For many who live in Jozi (a colloquial term for Johannesburg), the city is an entanglement of all these at once: optimism and desperation, possibility and disappointment, anticipation and despair. The paradoxes and ambiguities of living in a place like Johannesburg is, however, more acute for women and migrants, particularly those who are poor, Black, and sexual and gender non-conforming (Makandwa and Vearey 2017; Mbiyozo 2018; Walker 2017; Walker and Oliveira 2015).

The study that informs this chapter sought to better understand the lived experiences of women migrants in Johannesburg through their inclusion in all stages of the research process, particularly the production of knowledge about the issues that affect them (Walker and Oliveira 2020). In February 2017, the authors began working with a small group of women from across the African continent now living in Johannesburg on an arts-based project entitled Mwangaza Mama. The study involved partnership with the African Centre for Migration & Society[1] (ACMS), an interdisciplinary research center at the University of the Witwatersrand (Wits), and the Sophiatown

Community Psychological Services (SCPS), a local non-profit that offers various types of assistance to people living in and around the greater Johannesburg area.

Taking place over twenty-four months, Mwangaza Mama built on our previous experiences of using arts-based research strategies with diverse migrant communities (for example, see Oliveira 2016; Oliveira and Vearey 2017; Schuler and Oliveira 2018; Walker and Clacherty 2015) and forms part of the MoVE[2] (methods:visual:explore) project, an experimental research space at the ACMS that focuses on the development of arts-based methodologies (alongside more conventional study approaches) to explore (and elucidate) the lived experiences and needs of migrant groups that are typically excluded, under-represented, or misrepresented in research, policy, and public debates (Oliveira and Vearey 2018).

There were two main aims for Mwangaza Mama: first, to explore the everyday experiences of women migrants in Johannesburg; and second, to support the participants with creating their own visual and narrative outputs for public audiences. Arts-based methodologies, such as the textile work used in this study, "allow for journeys of self-discovery that are relational and not restricted by the limits of categories and labels" (Oliveira and Walker 2019: 35). When used responsibly and ethically, arts-based research strategies (e.g., photovoice, poetry, film) can provide participants an opportunity to actively engage in research, including controlling the ways they want to explore, portray, and represent their issues of concern and lived experiences (Capous-Desyllas and Morgaine 2018). In the context of feminist research and decolonizing research, which arts-based research can be situated, the focus is more than to "critically engage women's lived social realities with a view to change them for the better" (Kiguwa 2019: 220), there is also an acknowledgement that "researchers become part of circles of relations that are connected to one another and to which the researcher is accountable" (Chilisa 2012: 113).

Everyone who took part in Mwangaza Mama—participants, facilitators and researchers—were invited to share stories about their lives. Some spoke candidly about past and present circumstances whereas others preferred to listen; some created more than one visual and narrative story, but most produced one of each for public audiences. The inclusion of a visual approach in the project allowed for the telling of stories that are beyond the reach of words (Oliveira 2016) and the women's narratives poignantly illustrate the need for literary ways of knowing, which have always been critical to African feminist studies (Msimang 2019).

The Mwangaza Mama project workshops took place twice a month at one of two SCPS sites, and culminated in the production of three visual artifacts: two large collective quilts, each composed of individual quilt pieces made by everyone who took part (including the two authors) and one smaller quilt that features the project name and logo. Not only did the group spend many months stitching, gluing, and threading our individual quilt pieces (approximately 23 by 33 inches/59 by 84 centimeters), each of the seven participants also wrote one or two narrative stories about a topic or personal experience that they wanted to share with public audiences. A free downloadable eBook[3] that archives the project was also produced at the end of our time together.

The various artifacts that emerged out of Mwangaza Mama offer an important opportunity for audiences to reflect on the complex lives of women migrants, and they encourage us to consider the ways that stories are told and how different ways of telling might be used to create new forms of awareness and activism (Oliveira and Walker 2019).

All of the women who took part travelled to South Africa as asylum seekers after fleeing war, persecution, and other instabilities in their birth countries—Angola, Burundi, Rwanda, and the Democratic Republic of Congo (DRC). Although each crossed many borders in the hopes of finding safety and more secure lives in South Africa, only one had refugee status; the other six were waiting for decisions to be made on their asylum applications or were/are appealing rejections.[4] Six of the participants were mothers and single parents—the fathers of the children were either killed during conflict in their countries of origin, were in hiding, disappeared, or never around.

Similar to many foreign-born nationals in other parts of the world (Hiralal and Jinnah 2018), the Mwangaza Mama participants' everyday experiences were shaped by intersecting challenges, including difficulties accessing free public healthcare, formal employment, and schooling for their children; challenges that were amplified by ongoing xenophobic hostility and endemic levels of gender-based violence (Kihato 2009; Lefko-Everett 2007; Mbiyozo 2018; Hiralal and Jinnah 2018).

Caught between global and local circuits, and spaces of risk and opportunity, the Mwangaza Mama participants, through their movements and ambition, were often required to constantly negotiate (and renegotiate) patriarchy and ways of belonging. Like many other women in South Africa, our participants seemed to experience their lives as though they were suspended in time (Kihato 2013), what Loren Landau (2006: 125) refers to as existing in a "denationalized 'nowhereville.'"

The notion of "belonging" used in this chapter connotes not only the ways women migrants "root" themselves in a place, but also their positionality and understanding of how they felt they belonged (or not) in South Africa, and how belonging was negotiated in a context of hostilities and marginalization.

Migrant women's subjective lived experiences are shaped and influenced by their multiple identities (gender, race, class, sexuality, nationality, ethnicity, etc.) and the ways in which these identities interact and intersect across time and space (Matsuda et al. 2018). This hybridity can also be understood as living in the borderlands: "spaces that are not entirely physical nor completely abstract; spaces where multiple identities, histories, cultures, and ideologies overlap and collide" (Oliveira 2019: 525). As Chicano-feminist Gloria Anzaldúa (1987: i) explains, "Borderlands are present whenever two or more cultures edge each other, where people of different races occupy the same territory, where under, lower, middle and upper classes touch, where the space between two individuals shrinks with intimacy." For the Mwangaza Mama participants living in the borderlands was a spatial and temporal condition. Suffocated by unyielding physical, emotional, and psychological pressures and the need to constantly prove their legitimacy in order to gain rights to the city and society more broadly each had to strike a thorny balance between being visible enough to gain a footing in the city and invisible enough to elude persecution and harassment (Oliveira and Walker 2019). This in turn, added to the trauma that many had previously experienced in their birth countries and/or during their journeys to South Africa. As Caroline Kihato's (2007, 2009, 2013) seminal work shows us, women migrants clearly display agency, but their actions are often limited by structural economic, legal, and political forces, as well as by other non-material systems of regulation, such as gendered norms and cultural expectations.

This chapter seeks to understand the complex, ambiguous, and sometimes contradictory borderlands that women migrants in Johannesburg traverse and straddle. To do this, we draw on the stories shared and narrated during the project and examine four key intersecting issues: first, the difficulties of acquiring the required documentation to legally reside and work in South Africa; second, lack of employment and subsequent poverty; third, the challenges of accessing free public health care; and fourth, the hardship(s) of single parenting. These challenges have significant impact on migrant women's ability to "keep well" and their sense of well-being and belonging.

In this chapter well-being is conceptualized in line with the International Organization of Migration (IOM) as encompassing the following aspects: "community and social well-being (including safety satisfaction with public services and social connections), physical well-being and access to healthcare, career well-being (including employment and underemployment) and financial well-being" (Mazars 2013). This broad concept of well-being enables a holistic approach to health by opening up a space to explore the many complex and intersecting issues impacting the everyday lives of women and migrants. In particular, it shifts the focus from vulnerability due to pre-migration experiences of violence and loss to material, legal, and social contexts. A shift away from vulnerability also points to the importance of recognizing the role that societal and institutional contexts play in shaping migrant's lives. As Heide Castañeda and colleagues (2015: 376) explain, "factors such as employment, housing and living conditions, access to food and social services, and legal status are consequential for well-being." These factors contribute to the structural violence that deeply impact women's experiences. Structural violence refers to less visible, often indirect forms of harm that are experienced through societal structures, relationships, and ideologies (Bourgois 2009; De Maio 2015). Such normalized forms of violence are not only insidious; they can also negatively impact refugee women's sense of self, identity, and belonging. By moving beyond simplistic stereotypes and categories of vulnerability that are often applied to women and migrants, we show the need for a more nuanced understanding of what it means to survive and thrive in a new host country or city. And in so doing, we emphasize the importance for studies on health and well-being to engage with the complex lives of women migrants and their experiences of belonging, oppression, and perseverance.

Doing Research in a Precarious Context

The context of this research is the complex reality of post-apartheid South Africa, a country emerging out of the repression of apartheid (1948–1994) and the violence leading up to and through its transition to official democracy. Although classified as a middle-income country, South Africa is one of the most unequal places on the planet (Oxfam 2020). Despite this, South Africa continues to attract people seeking improved livelihoods and safe havens from across the globe, particularly the southern African region (Marnell, Oliveira, and Khan 2021; Palmary 2016). Contrary to popular perception, and in line with global trends, however, is the fact that international migrants in South Africa only constitute a small proportion of the population (Statistics South Africa 2015; UNDP 2017). According to the most reliable data available, South Africa's non-national population is only around 4 million, out of a total population of approximately 56 million (UNDP 2017). Far more numerically significant is internal migration, which is unevenly distributed across South Africa's nine national provinces (Statistics South Africa 2015). Yet, despite the relatively small number of foreign-born migrants, they are often blamed for South Africa's struggling education and public healthcare system, and lack of affordable housing and formal work opportunities (Hassim, Kupe, and Worby 2008; Makandwa and Vearey 2017). Similar to other contexts, these xenophobic myths have given rise to unrelenting discrimination, hostility, and harassment toward foreign-born nationals, including by government officials and ministers, in public hospitals and schools, and when dealing with law enforcement and Home Affairs officials (Crush and Peberdy 2018; Hassim et al. 2008).

Xenophobic violence in South Africa is particularly severe in Johannesburg—the financial epicenter of the continent. Built on cheap Black migrant labor after the discovery of gold in the 1800s, Johannesburg continues to attract people from both within and outside South Africa's national borders (Walker and Vearey 2019). Although many of the city's residents have been able to meet and surpass their livelihood expectations, the great majority live in poverty and struggle intensely to access basic services (Palmary, Hamber, and Núñez 2014). The severe inequality that characterizes the city is, however, typically felt and experienced more acutely for women migrants, many of whom are also heads of households and the sole providers of children.

Methodology

It was within this layered context that we sought to better understand the everyday experiences of women migrants through the use of participatory arts-based research approaches. Similar to other MoVE projects, our study incorporated creative study approaches with more traditional forms of inquiry, such as ethnography and narrative interviews.

The project took place from February 2017 to February 2019.[5] From the outset, we felt it was important to offer participants an opportunity to experiment with different ways of telling stories. During the initial months of the project, we invited the women to explore life stories through collage, drawing, writing, and simple body mapping exercises. Although they seemed to enjoy these activities, many also described their interest in (and experiences of) working with textiles. Almost all of the women learned to sew when they were children and continued making or altering their clothes. Many also embroidered and/or knitted with their families. It is perhaps not surprising then, that the women opted to work primarily with textile forms.

Several months after the project began; the group decided to work toward making a collective quilt that could be shared with public audiences. As Priscilla,[6] a woman from the Democratic Republic of the Congo (DRC)explained, "we have many stories to tell and it is important that we tell them ourselves." For the remaining eighteen months of our time together, each participant (plus the two of us) spent our time stitching, gluing, painting, and beading our individual quilt pieces, which were then stitched onto two large quilts.

In addition to creating visual stories for public audiences, the women also wrote one or two narrative stories that they wanted to share with various publics. Similar to the work and time that went into producing each quilt piece, the participants worked and re-worked their narrative stories, supporting one another in the process. During these moments, the women often gossiped about local happenings and at times, recounted tales of hope and horror, love and dreams, faith and betrayal. They also debated topics of interest to them and offered comfort to one another in times of distress. Reoccurring themes of group discussions tended to focus on the hardships that many experienced in the city, such as not being able to find formal employment, struggles getting their children a place in school, discrimination when seeking public health services, being robbed or assaulted, and loneliness. Questions of belonging also lingered. Not only did the women struggle to find a sense of place in Johannesburg, they also struggled to trust their own communities. As Kabibi from the DRC explained:

> Many of the South Africans don't like us and treat us badly but my own community, the Congolese people in South Africa and in the Congo are also not always the best. I told my kids that if something happens to me, they know where to go. They must go to Johanna [director of SCPS]. I don't want a Congolese taking care of them.

Although the women spent most of their time with migrants from their birth countries, the quote above show how simple notions of citizenship are inadequate when seeking to understand notions of belonging. Indeed, there were times the women spoke of the importance to have places where they could go to celebrate their cultural customs and traditions, such as churches, but at the same time spoke of their fellow migrants as those they mistrusted the most. Like all cities, Johannesburg is a tapestry of experiences and encounters; feeling a sense of belonging requires creativity and a constant mediation of ideas and ideologies, not only in terms of feeling part of a community or group but also in being able to survive in a city where borders, boundaries, and risks keep changing. Sarah Willen's (2012a) work exploring ideas of health-related deservingness with unauthorized im/migrants in Tel Aviv, describes this kind of creativity in terms of "trade-off/bargains" and calculated risks. Willen explains how im/migrants "actively activate a form of 'renegade morality' hinging not just on self-reliance but also on bending certain laws to serve objectives" (2012a: 819).

These objectives can include feeding themselves and their families, paying school fees, and accessing healthcare, all of which were daily struggles for the Mwangaza Mama participants.

Kihato (2013: 182) writes that "being un-rooted allows a critical distance and consciousness that resists being 'placed' somewhere, but allows migrant women to choose their place, depending on the circumstances." Negotiating these tensions was a central theme of our participant's stories and the ways they spoke of their everyday experiences, losses, gains, achievements, and tactics of survival. While the voices of women migrants remain largely absent in academic literatures and public debate, there is no doubt that their agency, tenacity, and actions shape and influence each and every space in which they live.

What's in a Name?

The title of the project—Mwangaza Mama—was chosen by the participants about halfway through our time together. Translated as "light," the Swahili word *mwangaza* has also been described by participants as meaning joy, love, caring, and togetherness. Although most of the women in the group were also mothers, the term "mama" in southern Africa is often used when referring to a woman, regardless of whether she is a parent or not. As Priscilla explained, "this name shows that our group is supportive to one another and to all women in the world." The title encapsulates much of what took place during the two years we spent together—the friendships that were built, the laughter and tears, and the caring during difficult times (Walker and Oliveira 2020)

Project workshops took place on Friday mornings, while most of the participants' children were at school. Often, they would begin with a communal breakfast because sharing meals is critical to establishing trust and rapport. Lunch and transportation to/from the workshop space was also provided. Although the women were able to communicate in basic English, we also used a translator. Pauline, a woman from the DRC who has lived in South Africa for more than five years, works for the SPCS and speaks French, Lingala, Swahili, and English. Balancing two roles, Pauline was both the project translator and a participant. Her presence in the group was fundamental to bridging language barriers and helping us better understand cultural nuances. Yet, as the workshops progressed, we also realized that words (in any oral language) are sometimes inadequate when seeking to convey embodied experiences.

Landscapes of Suffering

During workshops, the women often spoke of their lives "back home," of their journeys to South Africa, and of their deep longing for loved ones and places. They described their everyday experiences in Johannesburg and shed light on the physical, social, and imagined borders they encounter, traverse, and negotiate daily. Most recalled intense struggles of rejection and abuse, including gender-based violence, neglect, abandonment, and xenophobia, all of which led to increased marginalization and exclusion, in literal and figurative ways. While there certainly were moments during the workshop that the women's stories brought up deep pain and sorrow, there was also an unspoken acknowledgement and reminder in the group of the self-love, self-acceptance, and self-power that each woman cultivated and nourished.

Johanna Kistner, director of Sophiatown Community Psychological Services (SCPS), used the term "landscapes of suffering" in a reflection that she wrote for the project eBook to capture the multilayered experiences that many of the women she works with experience (Kistner 2015). Originally coined by a psychotherapist working with victims of political persecution in Zimbabwe, landscapes of suffering refer to the continuous nature of trauma. "It is a landscape in which people move from one experience of horror to another, in which the development of identities and social networks is continually disrupted and in which there are few, if any, safe spaces in which emotional refueling can take place" (Kistner 2015: 3). Chronic hardships and few safe spaces to "refuel" were reoccurring themes that emerged in our group discussions. The women often spoke of what they did to "keep going" and to "keep well" amid everyday challenges that required them to keep searching for hope, for a sign of change time and time again.

Ongoing experiences of suffering can also be understood through the concept of "extreme traumatization" (Becker 2004: 403), reflecting the many layers of violence and loss that often result in the "destruction of the individual, of his sense of belonging to society and of his social activities" (2004: 405). Noting the different conceptualizations of trauma and the developments within the discourses of trauma to looking at individual, collective, and social process, Becker locates "extreme traumatization" within specific cultural and political contexts. Trauma in this sense is entangled with the concept of well-being as fluid and constantly changing rather than as being an identified state or condition, as is common in traditional and medicalized approaches to health. While an in-depth exploration of the definitions of trauma is beyond the remit of this chapter, we aim to generate further questions about how it can be understood in specific social contexts and in relation to well-being. In particular, we draw on Bonnie Burstow's (2003) understanding of trauma as a form of "woundedness" and as a way of recognizing accounts of suffering as entangled and embedded with the contemporary realities of multiple forms of exclusion and "othering." As Burstow (2003: 1,302) suggests, "Trauma is not a disorder but a reaction to a kind of wound. It is a reaction to profoundly injurious events and situations in the real world and, indeed, to a world in which people are routinely wounded."

Notions of the wounded body have often been used to explore the significance of stigma and pain, and how trauma is transformed into a mode of survival and new sense of self. This is a critical intervention in that it powerfully shifts the focus from pure victimization and ideas of vulnerability to a recognition that tactics of survival and resistance can also weave through everyday life (Kihato 2007). Those who are wounded, suffer. But sometimes (often) wounded people also thrive.

In the context of the women discussed in this chapter, the wounded body is experienced through encounters with indirect and direct violence, which impact their health and sense of well-being as well as their coping mechanisms in everyday life. In the case of the Mwangaza Mamas, they are not only routinely wounded, their suffering is also routinely ignored, particularly in the very places and spaces of the city where they turn to for support, such as clinics and hospitals. Within this context, Willen (2012b: 808) reminds us, "unauthorised migrants face yet another form of exclusion, they are excluded not only from the political community, but also from the moral community of people whose lives, bodies, illnesses, and injuries are deemed worthy of attention, investment, or concern."

In this quote, Willen captures the multiple levels of exclusion that some migrants face as a result of their insecure documentation status, which is associated with a lack of rights and essentially renders them "illegal" or "unauthorized." An inherent aspect of discrimination is the process of "othering" whereby only certain people are seen as deserving, which can lead to increased experiences of harassment and abuse. In another article, Willen (2012a) complicates the notion of deservingness further by arguing the importance of focusing on the largely neglected views of those who are marginalized and objectified as "other." Through qualitative research, Willen (2012a: 819) shows how unauthorized migrants do not want to be perceived as "freeloading" and relying on handouts, but rather they "desire to be recognized as socially ratified persons capable of participating in everyday forms of reciprocity."

The following four key challenges that we present in this chapter reflect migrant women's attempts to participate in Johannesburg's social, economic, and political life; their attempts to "be seen" as individuals with rights, as city dwellers who belong, as human beings with needs and desires. In many ways, it is in their very attempts that the sheer brutality and battle of everyday life in Johannesburg is revealed. The idea of "being seen" is therefore paramount to having one's humanity recognized and respected.

Difficulties Acquiring the Required Documentation to Legally Reside and Work in the Country

> I am not a person . . . this small piece of paper . . . this is what I am. (Mary, 2017)

Of the many challenges described by the Mwangaza Mama participants, problems with documentation were often at the center. As previously mentioned, all of the women had lived in South Africa for a number of years, but only one had refugee status; the other six were waiting for decisions to be made on their asylum applications or were (are) appealing rejections. Unfortunately, this breakdown reflects a very real reality in South Africa, where 96 percent of asylum cases are rejected and the majority of asylum seekers wait countless years for resolution on their claims (Gandar 2019), which leaves many struggling to cope with severe insecurity and the risk of being detained and/or deported (Carciotto, Gastrow, and Johnson 2015).

In South Africa, those applying for refugee status, asylum seeker temporary permits, and permit renewal must report directly to the Department of Home Affairs (DHA) through one of five Refugee Reception Offices (RROs) located across the country (Carciotto et al. 2015). RROs are notoriously unable to accommodate the high numbers of people requiring assistance, particularly because two have been shut down and one has stopped accepting new applications. RROs are also plagued by corruption among those working at the offices, including clerks, interpreters, and security guards (Gandar 2019; Landau and Pampalone 2018). Asylum seekers can stand in queues for long hours, sometimes asked to pay a bribe just to be let inside the gate, only to be told that they have to come back another day (Amit 2015a). The gendered vulnerabilities of this process make it especially difficult for women supporting families and dependents because they can risk losing their employment if they run out of leave. Single mothers sometimes take children out of school so that they can travel with them and depending on circumstances, sleep in unsafe spaces near RRO offices in hopes of being first in line when they open[7] (Walker and Vearey 2019). This reality means that migrant women, through no fault of their own, often become undocumented. The consequences of not having documentation are far-reaching, such as being excluded from healthcare, education, employment, other forms of support, as well as the consequences of the psychological impact of uncertainty and fear (Mbiyozo 2018; Walker and Vearey 2019). In the quote below, Hannah, a middle-aged woman from Angola, highlights the frustrations and precarious context associated with not having a South African identity document:

> I have been living in South Africa for more than sixteen years, and I still don't have the right papers, only asylum permit which it not possible to do work. No one hired people like us. Now I am old. I used to work as a street vendor selling used clothing over there [*points*] but the police start to chase us away, saying they are cleaning the streets. But we are not rubbish. I had to stop because every time they come, I have to get my things and run. I started to have heart problems because of stress. Now the stress is different: no food.

While there were differences in the women's personal circumstances, all faced similar barriers to work and fears of arrest and deportation. During one of our sessions, we asked the women to list in order of significance the challenges they currently face in Johannesburg. Without hesitating, Priscilla answered, "paper, job, health, accommodation." The others nodded their heads in agreement and spoke at great length about the long hours they spent in lines only to be turned away or made to pay bribes to DHA security guards and/or immigration officials just to get their foot inside the building. The women talked about how they are always trying to "be seen" and recognized as more than a body in a queue, of being distinguishable from the hundreds of others, all of whom have their own stories and demands to be heard. As Mary from the DRC, noted, "they treat us worse than dogs."

One week, Kabibi, also from the DRC, arrived at the workshop and told the group that she had been mugged by a group of men who jumped out of a car, beat her up, and then drove off with her bag. She explained how the R2,000 (approximately $132) given to her by an anonymous donor to cover the costs of a chair in a hair salon so that she could begin earning money had been stolen. So had her phone and asylum papers. In recounting this traumatic experience Kabibi said,

> Even though I couldn't walk, everything was hurting . . . the next day I went back there to the place it happened. I checked for my bag in the bins and all over. I didn't find it, but I found my papers (asylum papers) . . . that was so lucky. If I lost those papers . . .

Kabibi's comments highlight the importance and significance of papers and what their physical presence represents. Kabibi had been badly beaten and was refused help by the public health care clinic. She was also ignored by the police when she went to report the case. But this was less important than the fact that her papers had been taken. While the bruises and the trauma of this incident were temporary, the loss of papers would have had a far greater impact on her everyday life. These papers, which could so easily be lost, vandalized, stolen, or torn affirmed Kibibi's rights to the city; they were her form of communication with those who challenged her existence and belonging; they held together the layers of her story—of how she came to be in Johannesburg and where she wanted to go. It was upon these papers that Kabibi's attempts to keep well were dependent.

The challenges of documentation had a huge impact on the women's sense of self, their well-being, and on their sense of (not) belonging in the city. Indeed, their very existence, at times, seemed hinged on a single piece of paper—a paper that granted them rights to work in South Africa, access to health care, accommodation, and education for their children.

This is why, Pauline, when told by a DHA official that her file had been lost and thus her asylum permit could not be renewed, refused to leave the office and demanded he find out what had happened. Pauline described standing inside and outside the official's office for an entire day. Even when the security guard tried to remove her, Pauline stood her ground and demanded that her story be heard. In her own words,

> I had arrived there the night before, waited in the long queue . . . no food . . . and then they tell you that the file is lost . . . No . . . I said to myself this can't be the end, they need to help me to find that file and so I stood and stayed there . . . that official got so angry . . . kept saying "I don't want to see your face" and asking "who is this woman that won't leave my office?" . . . but I stayed.

Pauline faced many tough experiences in life. She lost both of her parents as a young girl and brought up her siblings alone in extreme material poverty. Although Pauline felt fortunate to have a part time job with SCPS, life continued to be difficult. Not being able to renew her permit was in many ways just another struggle, except that so much of her life and well-being in South Africa was hinged on it.

While there are many such stories, those shared here show how documentation is simultaneously useless and vital. Useless because it is nearly impossible to find work with an asylum permit, and those lucky enough to possess it, are still often denied access to health care because they are "foreigners" and always treated as an "other" in their everyday lives. And vital because without these papers, they are even more invisible than ever. As Mary said, "I am not a person . . . this small piece of paper . . . this is what I am."

Lack of Employment and Subsequent Poverty

> There is no money for electricity, no sugar in the house, no Pampers [diapers] for my child . . . we are sitting in the dark and can't even make tea . . . (Priscilla, 2018)

Pauline was the only participant with a regular job. The others were all actively looking for work, but securing employment in South Africa is difficult even for most South Africans. Although the asylum seeker permit currently allows asylum seekers to be employed, many prospective employers discriminate and refuse them an opportunity to earn a living.[8] As the quote above by Priscilla illustrates, daily life situations were often desperate and often the women had to rely on the little support that NGOs and churches provided. While a few had qualifications they had obtained in their home countries, such as Priscilla, who was a qualified nurse, and Kabibi, a trained beautician, the nature of their temporary documentation status—and in Priscilla's case, South Africa's refusal to convert her DRC qualifications so that she could work—meant that most of the Mwangaza Mamas struggled intensely to meet their basic needs.

The women often compared their current situations in South Africa to "life before," aware that they had escaped war while at the same time they were depressed by the financial insecurity and violence they continued to face. For many, the suffering in South Africa was heightened, due in part to lack of support, distance from family and their land. And unrelenting xenophobia, as Kabibi explained,

> Back home I had respect . . . I came from a good family—we were not rich but we were comfortable you know. . . we went to school—these things were important . . . and then my husband was working and he was a professional man . . . but here I am asking for this small piece of bread, or sending the children to find something like, small, like some sugar or to borrow me something . . . and it's not nice . . . it makes you feel like all of that before is not you now . . . where is that respect?

The impact of financial poverty on the well-being of the women cannot be underestimated. The inability to meet basic needs coupled with the constant worry of eviction (accommodation was mostly a small section of a sub-divided room at extortionate rates) is extremely traumatic. All of the women found ways of earning small amounts of money through what they call "piece jobs" in South Africa—ad hoc work that is usually paid in cash, such as hand-washing clothes, braiding hair, making and selling cakes, and/or selling secondhand clothing on the street. Mary, a self-proclaimed "businesswoman" (and the only participant who did not have her children with her in South Africa) often traveled around the province looking for deals on food items and clothing that she could then sell in her neighborhood. Mary's tenacity, and her ability to move around without children, meant that she was often able to pay rent. Mary also lived in a more secure place than many of the other women, mostly because she only had to provide for herself.

There was one participant, Agape, who managed to start her own business. Although she faced daily violence in the inner city and relentless harassment by police, Agape kept a small stall open where she sold purses, bags, and other items by the Johannesburg main bus terminal. Similar to other foreign-born nationals, Agape was caught in a trap of not being able to get a business license because of her lack of documentation but she also needed to make money to survive. During a workshop, Agape described how she got around these barriers. She made friends with some homeless people and traders who lived and worked near her stall and gave them small gifts or money in trade for letting her know when the police were approaching. Although Agape lived with the constant fear of getting caught, she was also able to keep her shop going and make some money to support herself and her son.

Needing to be innovative and the willingness to take risks is, unfortunately, a reality for many people in the world. Although most of the Mwangaza Mama's found ways to earn an income, often through informal channels, their hustle was always precarious and dependent on a range of factors, such as health, documentation, childcare, and "the climate" of the city. Outbreaks of xenophobic violence make it very difficult (and dangerous) for non-nationals to go about their lives, and foreign-owned business are often the target of xenophobic destruction.

Challenges Accessing Free Public Healthcare

> It didn't even matter if the medication didn't work, just because he looked at me and saw me and spoke nicely to me asking me all about my life, I felt better. In the taxi on the way home, I felt better, and I hadn't even taken any medication. (Mary, 2017)

There are protective legislations, policies and international declarations that exist in South Africa to ensure access to primary public healthcare for all, regardless of nationality and documentation status. Pregnant and lactating women, and children under the age of six are also entitled to free care at all levels[9] (Walls et al. 2016). But in a struggling healthcare system where even South African nationals struggle to gain access, it is not uncommon that those without documentation are often asked to pay up front before seeing a doctor and receiving any treatment (Chekero and Ross 2017).

One of the most common discussions during the Mwangaza Mama workshops was on access to and treatment in the public healthcare system. Although the women's healthcare needs and those of their children varied (from seeking treatment for chronic stomach pain; a child born with hydrocephalus; injuries sustained when mugged, and the need for an abortion after rape) there are two key, interrelated issues that we would like to briefly highlight. One, is the impact of blocked access to health treatment, which can, of course, lead to ongoing illness or injury, and sometimes medical complications. The other is the psychological impact of "not being seen" and the ways this can add to additional layers of trauma.

The opening comment of this section by Mary was made during a workshop discussion about accessing healthcare and dealing with doctors. We share it because it captures the impact of these two intersecting issues. Mary explained how she had tried to see a doctor at a public health facility for nose bleeds. She described, "he [the doctor] sat and didn't look at me once . . . he asked me questions, but he never even looked at me. He was looking at his phone. He didn't check me, and he spoke in Zulu. I don't know Zulu." Mary compared this experience to when she saw a doctor in a private practice (facilitated by SCPS). "That doctor treated me like a human being," she said, "he checked everything." Understandably, Mary felt "seen" by this doctor because he physically examined her and listened to her concerns. These simple acts helped Mary feel better. Returning to Burstow's (2003) notion of trauma as a form of "woundedness" alongside Willen's comments about the exclusion of migrants from "the moral community of people whose lives, bodies, illnesses, and injuries are deemed worthy of attention, investment, or concern" (Willen 2012b: 808). It is clear from this example that the exclusion and "othering" that Mary felt possibly eroded her sense of belonging, and with it, her experiences of well-being.

A few weeks earlier, Priscilla described a healthcare encounter where she had gone to Baragwanath hospital (in Soweto) to pick up an appointment card to see a psychiatrist. The appointment had been arranged by SCPS and all that Priscilla needed was the card so that she knew when to attend. On arrival, Priscilla asked a nurse where she could collect the card, and the nurse turned to her and said (as recounted by Priscilla):

> You need to see a psychiatrist? For what? Trauma? You don't have trauma—I have seen trauma before. You are not traumatized. If you have problems with your husband, go sort it out, don't bring it here. We are not for you people to bring your problems.

What followed, according to Priscilla, was an onslaught of abuse from the nurse that left her in tears. Another nurse tried to apologize and a security guard tried to intervene. But Priscilla was unable to get her appointment card, the only route through which she might access crucial health care to ensure her mental and physical health, as well as her overall well-being, was blocked.

The kind of hostility that Priscilla described seems to be influenced by common and prevailing perceptions within South African policy-making debates, everyday discussions, and popular media that foreign-born migrants, and especially pregnant women, come to South Africa specifically to gain access to healthcare and thus are often the scapegoats for the defunct healthcare system (Machiwenyika and Munatswa 2020).

A similar rhetoric is also evident in questions that are often raised about the health of those who move and its impact on the health of the local population (Vearey and Nunez 2011) For example, despite widespread acknowledgement that "healthy migration is good for development" (Vearey 2014: 663) and findings showing that migrants tend to be healthier than those they leave behind and healthier than host populations (Vearey 2010), cross-border migrants are often perceived as disease carriers (Chekero and Ross 2017; Walker 2017). This notion was reflected in some of the stories participants recounted, particularly when describing a negative encounter with a medical professional. As Agape said, "the nurse said to me that we are the problem because we come here and cause troubles . . . bring disease and problems . . . and that South Africa can't look after us."

In these examples, both Agape and Priscilla show that despite inclusive laws and policies, in practice, there are tensions that can severely impact a person's experience of well-being and care (see also Coovadia et al. 2009; Makandwa and Vearey 2017).

The Hardship(s) of Single Parenting

> You think coming here things will be easier . . . like this is a better place to be, and we can be safe and get help . . . but then it's not like that. And for the kids, this is not a good place . . . if we had money, if I could get a good job I could look after them. . . (Kabibi, 2018)

Parenting and being single mothers were issues that were readily discussed during the project. Very real challenges of bringing up young children alone in a context of poverty, little stability, without regular income, persistent marginalization and violence were immense. These realities often left the women questioning their ability to care for their children. In the literature, when motherhood is reflected in relation to migration and migrant women, it is often shaped by a focus on either the "transnational mother" who is physically distant from her child(ren) and sending remittances home, or the "victim mother" in a refugee camp and vulnerable (Walker, Vearey, and Nencel 2017). There has been little exploration of migrant women who have their children with them, and what it means to provide while dealing with multiple, often violent challenges in present and past circumstances. Yet, for the Mwangaza Mama participants, the responsibility of providing for children, not only financially but physically and emotionally as well, wove through almost everything they spoke of.

Agape, described the challenges of being a single parent as "sometimes making you sick with worry." Agape lost her father and almost all of her siblings in the Rwandan genocide and fled the country as a teenager after being raped by a police officer. By the time she arrived at the central Johannesburg train station, Agape was not only heavily pregnant but also destitute and unable to speak the local languages to ask for help. Agape eventually received some help from a fellow Rwandan after she heard him speaking Swahili and was directed to a women's shelter where she was given temporary accommodation until her child was born. Although Agape has since managed to provide for her child by selling fashion items at her shop, she often spoke of the loneliness of parenting alone. Without family around, Agape was the sole provider for her son. She did not have someone to help care for him while she was at work. As a new mom, Agape also missed her own mother with whom she has not had contact since leaving Rwanda. The fear and loneliness of being a single parent, and her longing for her mom, weighed heavily on Agape and the ways in which she experienced life and the city.

When speaking of motherhood and single parenting in the context of the Mwangaza Mama project, it is critical to point out that it is not about saying that someone was a "bad" or incapable mother. In South Africa (and elsewhere), there are common negative assumptions made about migrant women with children, ranging from the idea that women have children simply to access documentation to having children in order to gain support from the state, which in reality does not exist in South Africa. For us, attention to motherhood and single parenting is all about highlighting the gendered nature of migration and the too-often neglected torment that poor women migrants who are single parents face.

A tragic example of this torment was shared by Celine, a mother to three children from Burundi who was present at the very start of Mwangaza Mama. One day she arrived at the group in crisis. She looked visibly exhausted and said she was "giving up." Through tears, Celine described how she had spent the previous might searching for rat poison. In her own words, Celine said, "I wish I could die. At least then someone would have to take care of my kids." Some weeks later, Celine informed us that she was leaving the group because she had decided to travel to a neighboring country to buy used clothing to sell in Johannesburg. Although we expressed concern, mostly because her documentation was not finalized and she was leaving her children behind, Celine was adamant that this was her only option. Celine's husband had recently returned to Johannesburg after disappearing for some months, and she thought he could care for the children. So she was not abandoning them; she was searching for another way. In the weeks before she left, we watched her get thinner and thinner. The family had no food and what she was given by the NGO she fed the children. Celine had hit her breaking point. Burned out and stressed out by the expectations associated with being a mother who felt like she had nothing left to give, Celine she was trying to keep going so that she could "keep well" (Walker 2018).

Celine never returned to Johannesburg. And while there probably were many complex reasons that led to her decision to leave in the first place, the sheer level of exhaustion and isolation that Celine experienced cannot be ignored. For women who are traumatized, women who are expected to provide as mothers, with little (if any) support while at the same time in the grip of multiple forms of violence, there often feels like there are few alternatives (Walker 2018).

Keeping Well in the City

The four main issues that we describe in this chapter (difficulties acquiring the documentation required to legally reside and work in South Africa; lack of formal employment opportunities; challenges accessing free public healthcare; and hardship(s) of single parenting) highlight the immense challenges that many people face in Johannesburg. These experiences have a massive impact on the well-being of migrant women. From the participant's stories, it is clear that the demands and responsibilities of providing as mothers and the challenges of caring for themselves and their children when met with dire poverty, persistent gender-based violence and brutal xenophobia compromise what they can do. Yet, despite the fact that many (like Celine) frequently expressed a desire to give up, none did. Week after week, the Mwangaza Mama participants came back to our group, often saying "we are still trying; we are still here." Although they were realistic and knew that their challenges were not going to disappear or that life would suddenly become easy, all hung on tightly to the hope that things could improve one day. There were moments during the workshop where the women witnessed an improvement. Whether it was Agape's efforts to keep her shop open or Mary's experience of being properly seen and cared for by a doctor or Pauline's victory at the Department of Home Affairs, these small wins reminded the women that they could push forward, they have agency, and, despite the many challenges they face, efforts to keep going are ultimately worth it.

As Kihato (2007) makes poignantly clear, migrant women's lives are shaped by the city, but in turn they also change the city. But in order to gain a nuanced understanding of migrant women's lives we must search for alternative ways of seeing and understanding lived experiences and circumstances. Kihato's argument that there is a need to collapse the binary conceptual frames that depict women as either victims or victors is also critical. Drawing from interviews with women migrants from various African countries, now living in Johannesburg, Kihato argues that there is a need for balance in the ways that migrant women are represented. As she explains, "while women do have mechanisms for navigating difficult social situations, their well-being should not be that of individual responsibility, but a communal one as well" (Kihato 2007: 105). Similarly, an understanding of the everyday lives of the Mwangaza Mama participants also demands a balancing of the harsh and often violent realities that are shaped by the challenges of being a single parent, of accessing documentation, of poverty, and of access to healthcare. The Mwangaza Mama's embodied experiences of agency and victimhood, of vulnerability and strength are complexly intertwined and as such, demand new ways of thinking and new approaches to understand well-being and belonging. As Elizabeth Marino and Heather Lazrus go on to explain in greater detail in the following chapter, increased attention to the lived experiences of migrants is necessary for those seeking to gain a more holistic (and nuanced) understanding of migration pressures, at the systemic, community, and individual levels. The development and implementation of methodologies that open (or at least try to open) the practical and intellectual space for reflexivity on behalf of everyone involved—participants, researchers, and wider publics—is also key to confronting and debunking categories of "victimhood" that too often obscure (rather than reveal) migrants' agency and tenacity, as well as the structures that negatively impact their lives.

Conclusion

This chapter highlighted the various challenges, and forms of discrimination and abuse that asylum-seeking and refugee women face while living in Johannesburg and the ways they impact upon and shape their experiences of well-being and belonging.

Difficulties accessing documentation and free public health care, challenges finding employment and subsequently living in poverty, and the hardships of parenting alone weave into an overarching narrative of the daily challenges faced by non-nationals in South Africa, a place where protective legislations, policies, and international declarations to protection and rights are easily ignored (Amit 2015b; Amit and Gastrow 2015; Mthembu-Salter et al. 2014). Although there is growing attention and debate on migrants and their health and well-being in South Africa, there remains a gap in terms of understanding and engaging with their everyday realities, especially the intersecting nature of what it means to be a migrant, a woman and a mother trying to keep well and "be seen" in a complicated city. These layered realities reflect the precarious context of life, particularly for those who have experienced hardship and trauma when fleeing their birth countries, which intensifies the struggle to maintain a sense of well-being in South Africa. As this chapter has shown, Mwangaza Mama's narratives often focused on experiences of discriminatory, abusive, and malicious treatment toward them. The women expressed a range of emotions throughout the project, including sentiments of rage, disappointment, and anger. They spoke candidly of their frustrations and hardships and of being disrespected by South Africans, and at times, their families and communities. Underscoring these narratives, however, were demands to be seen and be treated differently and examples of the ways they resisted (sometimes aligned with) gendered, cultural norms and expectations. Human experiences are complex, and the stories shared by the women who took part in Mwangaza Mama show us the importance of recognizing multilayered and sometimes contradictory and ambiguous experiences. These are experiences that do not fit easily into categories of victimhood/vulnerability or resilience and defy simple interpretations that are often sought after by those looking to understand and/or assist; a migrant woman may show tenacity and strength and at the same time feel vulnerable, she may experience love and desire simultaneous with hate and despair. In this way, we can on one level move beyond linear understandings and recognize migrant women as layered, complex beings. But to take this further, we can also reflect on the lives of women who are pushed into the margins because of their race, sexuality, and socio-economic realities, and subsequently, we can demand a more complex and urgent recognition of their needs and experiences. As Willen and Cook (in the preceding chapter) explain, we ought to pay more attention to how "undeservingness" is "reckoned with both in relation to and from the perspectives of those most directly affected." The lived experiences of the Mwangaza Mama women powerfully show that self-recognition and self-worth are not synonymous with the ways they were treated. But the ways they were treated had a direct impact on their everyday experiences. How we speak and use terms to describe people matters. Resisting the temptation to simplify while also embracing complexity is, therefore, essential in social justice work, particularly in public health efforts seeking to humanize and push for change.

Rebecca Walker is a Research Associate with the African Centre for Migration & Society (ACMS), The University of the Witwatersrand, Johannesburg. With a background in social anthropology, Rebecca has worked broadly on issues related to gender, migration and health with a specific focus on the experiences of asylum-seeking and refugee women in South Africa. Her recent work has looked at access to health care and migration and mental health in the context of displacement and forced migration. Rebecca has published widely across academic and non-academics spaces and consults for a number of local and international organizations.

Elsa Oliveira is a postdoctoral researcher and a National Research Foundation (NRF) fellow at the African Centre for Migration and Society (ACMS), Wits University, where she also co-coordinates the MoVE (method.visual.explore) project. Elsa has a PhD in Migration and Displacement and works in the areas of gender, sexualities, well-being, and informal livelihoods. With a commitment to social justice, Elsa often uses participatory community-based research strategies to better understand the lived experiences of migrant women, men, and transgender persons in South Africa and the ways research can be used to support public engagement. Elsa has published widely in both popular and academic spaces.

Notes

1. "The African Centre for Migration & Society." *ACMS*. Retrieved 7 January 2022 from http://www.migration.org.za/.
2. "MoVE method:visual:explore." *Migration and Health Project, Southern Africa*. Retrieved 7 January 2022 from https://www.mahpsa.org/arts-based-research/move/
3. "Mwangaza Mama." *Migration and Health Project, Southern Africa*. Retrieved 7 January 2022 from https://www.mahpsa.org/mwangaza-mama/
4. At the time of publication, the participants are still waiting for resolution on their documentation status. This has been delayed further by the impact of the Covid-19 pandemic which led to the closure of the Department of Home Affairs and increased the backlog of applications and appeals.
5. The study received ethical approval (H16/11/42) from the University of Witwatersrand (Wits) Research Ethics Committee (nonmedical) and forms part of a postdoctoral study at the ACMS and was funded through a Life in the City grant from the Wits School of Governance. Security at the Margins (SeaM), a collaborative project involving partnership with Wits University and the University of Edinburgh also provided funding.
6. All of the names used in this paper are pseudonyms we chose for the participants. Although all of the women selected the names they wanted to use in their public outputs, we felt that it was important to change these as an additional step to protect their anonymity.
7. A recent research report shows how the decisions made by the DHA as well as the refusal to comply with various court orders to reopen RROs have had a disproportionate impact on women, children and sexual and gender minorities within the asylum-seeking population in South Africa (Gandar 2019).
8. Proposed amendments to the Refugee Act would remove this right and restrict the movements of asylum seekers and restrict their ability to "self-settle" in South Africa.
9. As a member state to The World Health Assembly (WHA), South Africa is constitutionally mandated to ensure access to health care for internal and cross-border migrant populations in line with the 2008 WHA resolution (Walls et al. 2016) In addition, the

South African Constitution (1996), as interpreted within the National Health Act (The Republic of South Africa 2003), guarantees rights to access health care for everyone in South Africa and also provides for the right to dispute resolution (Makandwa and Vearey 2017).

References

Amit, Roni. 2015a. *Queue Here for Corruption: Measuring Irregularities in South Africa's Asylum System*. Pretoria: Lawyers for Human Rights.

———. 2015b. "The Expansion of Illegality: Immigration Detention in South Africa." In *Immigration Detention: The Migration of a Policy and Its Human Impact*, ed. Amy Nethery and Stephanie J. Silverman, 147–55. London: Routledge.

Amit, Roni, and Vania Gastrow. 2015. *Lawless Regulation: Government and Civil Society Attempts at Regulating Somali Informal Trade in Cape Town*. Johannesburg: University of the Witwatersrand.

Anzaldúa, Gloria E. 1987. *Borderlands/La Frontera: The New Mestiza*. 4th ed. San Francisco, CA: Aunt Lute Books.

Becker, David. 2004. "Dealing with the Consequences of Organised Violence in Trauma Work." In *Transforming Ethnopolitical Conflict: The Berghof Handbook*, ed. Alex Austin, Martina Fischer, and Norbert Ropers, 403–20. Wiesbaden: VS Verlag für Sozialwissenschaften. https://doi.org/10.1007/978-3-663-05642-3_19.

Bourgois, Philippe. 2009. "Recognizing Invisible Violence: A Thirty-Year Ethnographic Retrospective." In *Global Health in Times of Violence*, ed. Barbara Rylko-Bauer, Linda Whiteford, and Paul Farmer, 17–40. Santa Fe, NM: School for Advanced Research Press.

Burstow, Bonnie. 2003. "Toward a Radical Understanding of Trauma and Trauma Work." *Violence against Women* 9(11): 1293–317.

Capous-Desyllas, Moshula, and Karen. Morgaine, eds. 2018. *Creating Social Change through Creativity: Anti-Oppressive Arts-Based Research Methodologies*. London: Palgrave Macmillan.

Carciotto, Sergio, Vanya Gastrow, and Corey Johnson. 2015. *The Impact of Curtailing Asylum Seekers' Right to Work in South Africa*. Cape Town: Scalabrini Institute for Human Mobility in Africa. Retrieved 7 January 2022 from https://sihma.org.za/reports/manufacturing-illegality-the-impact-of-curtailing-asylum-seekers-right-to-work-in-south-africa.

Castañeda, Heide. Seth M. Holmes, Daniel S. Madrigal, Maria-Elena DeTrinidad Young, Naomi Beyeler, and James Quesada. 2015. "Immigration as a Social Determinant of Health." *Annual Review of Public Health* 36: 375–92.

Chekero, Tamuka, and Fiona C. Ross. 2017. "'On Paper' and 'Having Papers': Migrants Navigating Medical Xenophobia and Obstetric Rights in South Africa." *Somatosphere: Science, Medicine, and Anthropology*, 25 October. Retrieved 6 January 2022 from http://somatosphere.net/2017/on-paper.html/.

Chilisa, Bagele. 2012. *Indigenous Research Methodologies*, 2nd ed. Los Angeles, CA: SAGE publications. Retrieved 7 January 2022 from https://www.vitalsource.com/za/products/indigenous-research-methodologies-bagele-chilisa-v9781544391496.

Coovadia, Hoosen. Rachel Jewkes, Peter Barron, David Sanders and Diane McIntyre. 2009. "The Health and Health System of South Africa: Historical Roots of Current Public Health Challenges." *Lancet* 374(9692): 817–34.

Crush, Jonathan, and Sally Peberdy. 2018. *Criminal Tendencies: Immigrants and Illegality in South Africa*. Southern African Migration Programme (SAMP). Retrieved 7 January 2022 from https://www.africaportal.org/publications/criminal-tendencies-immigrants-and-ille gality-south-africa/.

De Maio, Fernando. 2015. "Paul Farmer: Structural Violence and the Embodiment of Inequality." In *The Palgrave Handbook of Social Theory in Health, Illness and Medicine*, ed. Fran Collyer, 675–90. London: Palgrave Macmillan UK.

Gandar, Sally. 2019. *'They Treated Me as If I Was Nothing': Research Report on the Gendered Impact of the Decision to Close the Cape Town Refugee Reception Office*. Sonke Gender Justice, July 2019: https://genderjustice.org.za/publication/they-treated-me-as-if-i-was-nothing/

Hassim, Shireen, Tawana Kupe, and Eric Worby, eds. 2008. *Go Home or Die Here: Violence, Xenophobia and the Reinvention of Difference in South Africa*. Johannesburg: Wits University Press.

Hiralal, Kalpana, and Zaheera Jinnah, eds. 2018. *Gender and Mobility in Africa: Borders, Bodies and Boundaries*. Cham: Palgrave Macmillan.

Kiguwa, Peace. 2019. "Feminist Approaches: An Exploration of Women's Gendered Experiences." In *Transforming Research Methods in the Social Sciences: Case Studies from South Africa*, eds. Sumaya Laher, Angelo Flynn, and Sherianne Kramer, 220–235. Johannesburg: WITS University Press.

Kihato, Caroline W. 2007. "Invisible Lives, Inaudible Voices? The Social Conditions of Migrant Women in Johannesburg." *African Identities* 5(1): 89–110.

———. 2009. "Migration, Gender and Urbanisation in Johannesburg." Ph.D. dissertation. Pretoria, South Africa: University of South Africa.

———. 2013. *Migrant Women of Johannesburg: Everyday Life in an In-Between City*. New York: Palgrave Macmillan.

Kistner, Johanna. 2015. "From Personal Tragedy to Global Responsibility: Re-politicizing Trauma Work in an African Context." *AIR Thoughts* 2: 1–6. Retrieved 7 January 2022 from https://sophiatowncounselling.files.wordpress.com/2018/02/from-personal-tragedy-to-global-responsibility.pdf

Landau, Loren B. 2006. "Transplants and Transients: Idioms of Belonging and Dislocation in Inner-City Johannesburg." *African Studies Review* 49(2): 125–45.

Landau, Loren. 2018. "Displacement and the Pursuit of Urban Protection: Forced Migration, Fluidity, and Global Cities." In *Forced Migration: Current Issues and Debates*, ed. Alice Bloch and Giorgia Dona. London: Routledge.

Landau, Loren, and Tanya Pampalone, eds. 2018. *I Want to Go Home Forever: Stories of Becoming and Belonging in South Africa's Great Metropolis*. Johannesburg: Witts University Press.

Lefko-Everett, Kate. 2007. *Voices from the Margins: Migrant Women's Experiences in Southern Africa*, no. 46, Migration Policy Series. Waterloo, ON: The Southern African Migration Project.

Machiwenyika, Moffat R., and Elvis T. Munatswa. 2020. "The Paradox of Free Access to Maternal Health: The Twofold Narrative of Pregnant Migrant Women in Johannesburg." *Southern African Journal of Public Health Incorporating Strengthening Health Systems* 4(1): 4–9.

Makandwa, Tackson, and Jo Vearey. 2017. "Giving Birth in a Foreign Land: Exploring the Maternal Healthcare Experiences of Zimbabwean Migrant Women Living in Johannesburg, South Africa." *Urban Forum* 28(1): 75–90.

Marnell, John, Elsa Oliveira, and Gabriel Hoosain Khan. 2021. "'It's about Being Safe and Free to Be Who You Are': Exploring the Lived Experiences of Queer Migrants, Refugees and Asylum Seekers in South Africa." *Sexualities* 24(1–2): 86–110.

Matsuda, Mari, Charles Lawrence, Richard Delgado, and Kimberlé Williams Crenshaw. 2018. *Words that Wound: Critical Race Theory, Assaultive Speech, and the First Amendment.* New York: Routledge.

Mazars, Céline. 2013. "The Well-Being of Economic Migrants in South Africa: Health, Gender and Development." *International Organization for Migration*, Working Paper for the World Migration Report 2013.

Mbiyozo, Aimée-Noël. 2018. "Gender and Migration in South Africa: Talking to Women Migrants." Institute for Security Studies, Southern Africa Report 16.

Msimang, Sisonke. 2019. *Always Another Country: A Memoir of Exile and Home.* New York: Jonathan Ball.

Mthembu-Salter, Gregory, Roni Amit, Chandre Gould, and Loren Landau. 2014. "Counting the Cost of Securitising South Africa's Immigration Regime." Brighton, UK: Migrating Out of Poverty Research Programme Consortium, University of Sussex. Working Paper 20.

Oliveira, Elsa. 2016. "Empowering, Invasive or a Little Bit of Both? A Reflection on the Use of Visual and Narrative Methods in Research with Migrant Sex Workers in South Africa." *Visual Studies* 31(3): 260–78.

———. 2019. "The Personal Is Political: A Feminist Reflection on a Journey into Participatory Arts-Based Research with Sex Worker Migrants in South Africa." *Gender & Development* 27(3): 525–40.

Oliveira, Elsa, and Jo Vearey. 2017. "Beyond the Single Story: Creative Research Approaches with Migrant Sex Workers in South Africa." *Families, Relationships and Societies* 6(2): 317–21.

———. 2018. "Making Research and Building Knowledge with Communities: Examining Three Participatory Visual and Narrative Projects with Migrants Who Sell Sex in South Africa." In *Creating Social Change through Creativity: Anti-Oppressive Arts-Based Research Methodologies*, ed. Moshoula Capous-Desyllas and Karen Morgaine, 265–87. Cham: Springer International Publishing.

Oliveira, Elsa, and Rebecca Walker, eds. 2019. *Mwangaza Mama: A Participatory Arts-Based Research Project.* Johannesburg, South Africa: MoVE and ACMS, University of the Witwatersrand. Retrieved 7 January 2022 from https://issuu.com/move.methods.visual .explore/docs/mwangaza_mama_ebook.

Oxfam. 2020. *Reclaiming Power: Womxn's Work and Income Inequality in South Africa.* November 2020: https://www.oxfam.org.za/wp-content/uploads/2020/11/oxfam-sa-inequality-in-south-africa-report-2020.pdf

Palmary, Ingrid 2016. "The Normalization of Violence: Gender, Sexuality and Asylum." In *Gender, Sexuality and Migration in South Africa: Governing Morality*, ed. Ingrid Palmary, 31–52. Cham: Palgrave MacMillan.

Palmary, Ingrid, Brandon Hamber, and Lorena Núñez, eds. 2014. *Healing and Change in the City of Gold: Case Studies of Coping and Support in Johannesburg.* Cham: Palgrave MacMillan.

Schuler, Greta, and Elsa Oliveira. 2018. "'Something about Us for Us': Exploring Ways of Making Research with Sex Workers in South Africa.'" In *Routledge International Handbook of Sex Industry Research*, ed. Susan Dewey, Isabel Crowhurst, and Chimaraoke Izugbara. New York: Routledge.

Statistics South Africa. 2015. *Census 2011: Population Dynamics in South Africa.* Pretoria: Statistics South Africa.

The Republic of South Africa. 2003. *National Health Act, 2003 (Act No. 61 of 2003).* Cape Town: The Republic of South Africa.
UNDP (United Nations Development Programme). 2017. *Inequality-Adjusted Human Development Index.* New York: UNDP.
Vearey, J., and L. Nunez. 2011. *Towards Improving Formed Migrant Access to Health and Psychosocial Rights in Urban South Africa - a Focus on Johannesburg* (Migration Issue brief #8): https://media.africaportal.org/documents/brief_8_migration.pdf.
Vearey, Jo. 2010. "Hidden Spaces and Urban Health: Exploring the Tactics of Rural Migrants Navigating the City of Gold." *Urban Forum* 21(1): 37–53.
———. 2014. "Healthy Migration: A Public Health and Development Imperative for South (ern) Africa." *South African Medical Journal* 104(10): 663–64.
Walker, R., and J. Vearey. 2019. *Gender, Migration and Health in SADC: A Focus on Women and Girls. Issue Brief 1 Key Findings.* Johannesburg, South Africa: Sonke Gender Justice.
Walker, Rebecca. 2017. "Selling Sex, Mothering and 'Keeping Well' in the City: Reflecting on the Everyday Experiences of Cross-Border Migrant Women Who Sell Sex in Johannesburg." *Urban Forum* 28(1): 59–73.
———. 2018. "Migrant Mothers and the Burden of Care: Reflections from Johannesburg." *Families, Relationships and Societies* 7(2): 349–53.
Walker, Rebecca, Jo Vearey, and Lorraine Nencel. 2017. "Negotiating the City: Exploring the Intersecting Vulnerabilities of Non-National Migrant Mothers Who Sell Sex in Johannesburg, South Africa." *Agenda* 31(1): 91–103.
Walker, Rebecca, and Glynis Clacherty. 2015. "Shaping New Spaces: An Alternative Approach to Healing in Current Shelter Interventions for Vulnerable Women in Johannesburg." In *Healing and Change in the City of Gold: Case Studies of Coping and Support in Johannesburg*, ed. Ingrid Palmary, Brandon Hamber, and Lorena Núñez, 31–58. Cham: Palgrave MacMillan.
Walker, Rebecca, and Elsa Oliveira. 2015. "Contested Spaces: Exploring the Intersections of Migration, Sex Work and Trafficking in South Africa." *Graduate Journal of Social Science* 11(2): 129–513.
———. 2020. "A Creative Storytelling Project with Women Migrants in Johannesburg, South Africa." *Studies in Social Justice* 14(1): 188–209.
Walls, Helen L., Jo Vearey, Moeketsi Modisenyane, Candice M. Chetty-Makkan, Salome Charalambous, Richard D. Smith, and Johanna Hanefield. 2016. "Understanding Healthcare and Population Mobility in Southern Africa: The Case of South Africa." *South African Medical Journal* 106(1): 14–155.
Willen, Sarah S. 2012a. "How Is Health-Related 'Deservingness' Reckoned? Perspectives from Unauthorized Im/Migrants in Tel Aviv." *Social Science & Medicine* 74(6): 812–21.
———. 2012b. "Migration, 'Illegality,' and Health: Mapping Embodied Vulnerability and Debating Health-Related Deservingness." *Social Science & Medicine* 74(6): 805–11.

3

Migration or Forced Displacement?

The Complex Choices of Climate Change and Disaster Migrants in Shishmaref, Alaska, and Nanumea, Tuvalu

Elizabeth Marino and Heather Lazrus

Three decades of research on climate change and climate change-related disasters have suggested that human migration and forced displacement will be a critical, if complex, outcome of anthropogenic climate change (IOM 2008, 2011; Lazrus 2012a; Marino 2012, 2013; N. Myers 1993; Oliver-Smith 2013). In 1990, the Intergovernmental Panel on Climate Change claimed that human migration may be the most significant outcome of anthropogenic climate change (IPCC 1990) and subsequently researchers have demonstrated a lack of political safety nets and governance structures equipped to handle communities fleeing from increasingly uninhabitable locations (Bronen 2009, 2011; Maldonado et al. 2013; Warner 2010). While the nuances of these moves are only beginning to be understood in detail, human populations will experience anthropogenic climate change through processes of slow-onset and rapid-onset hazards and other environmental changes. As a result, people are likely to relocate in order to avoid catastrophe.

Disaster anthropologists understand that disasters and the outcomes of disasters are primarily socially constructed circumstances (Button 2010; Oliver-Smith 1996) expressed when ecological events expose pre-existing socioeconomic vulnerabilities (Oliver-Smith 2004). Because of this, we can expect that climate change-related disasters will affect vulnerable populations first and more significantly than other populations (Crate 2011; Lazrus 2012a). The adaptive (systematic decisions that improve or maintain social conditions in response to risk) or coping (improvisational decisions that allow for survival but may deteriorate social conditions) (Smit and Wandel 2006; for full discussion, see Oliver-Smith 2013) choices available to populations directly experiencing climate change outcomes may be influenced and restricted by other pressures. Thus, decisions about migration and relocation in response to risk may be influenced by other migration pressures on the ground, such as economic need, development policy, and rural infrastructure deterioration that are already engines of urbanization globally. In other words, it is likely that hazardous events, which drive migration and displacement, will interact with other migration pressures to create complex, multilayered scenarios within which individuals, families, and communities make decisions. The movement of people, therefore, may not easily fit into the dichotomy of "forced displacement" resulting from immediate risk or "voluntary migration" resulting from individual or family preference and decision making, but may be a complex product of both.

While there are a handful of ethnographic case studies emerging about how local populations experience migration pressures as an outcome of climate change and natural hazards (Birk and Rasmussen 2014; Black, Kniveton, and Schmidt-Verkerk 2011; Farbotko and Lazrus 2012; Marino 2012, 2013; Massey, Axinn, and Ghimire 2010), it remains unclear how disaster-related migration pressures interact with other migration pressures in the lived experience of people on the ground (Nurse et al. 2014). Likewise, it is uncertain how vulnerability interacts with migration pressures in climate change scenarios and whether migration decisions in the event of a disaster are made under duress and constrained inventories of possibility (forced displacement) or are actually a locally preferred mechanism of adaptation and risk mitigation among populations exposed to ecological shift (voluntary migration as successful adaptation). Do people exposed to risk via disasters and climate change related disasters see moving as a viable adaptation strategy or is movement actively resisted and made as a decision of last resort? Clearly, the answer will differ across geographic place, time, and personal contexts as cultures, economic opportunities, and political backdrops differ significantly from place to place, community to community, and individual to individual; however, evidence suggests that marginalized populations are more at risk of migration following a disaster than other groups (Hunter 2005; C. Myers, Slack, and Singelmann 2008). What remains missing in the literature is an assessment of how climate- and hazard-related migration pressures interact with other migration pressures and adaptation options on the ground. This remains true in spite of a growing body of theoretical writing and policy research on the subject of climate change and migration (Black et al. 2011).

What we find, using ethnographic assessment, is that the drivers of migration are less distinct on the ground and the differences between forced displacement and voluntary migration can blur in the lives of individuals. When a young, college-educated resident of Shishmaref decides to move to Anchorage, in part because there are no housing options available to her outside of the floodplain, is this an example of global urbanization trends or is this forced displacement linked to climate change?

When a critical number of Tuvalu-ans leave an island community for work in New Zealand and crucial infrastructure is no longer maintained, is the resulting vulnerability to changing precipitation patterns due to development decisions or climate change impacts? When an extremely, and increasingly, rural village is at risk from climate change-related flooding, does it still merit protection and maintenance from the state?

In this chapter, we use the case studies from Shishmaref, Alaska, and Nanumea, Tuvalu to examine how climate change hazards (primarily coastal flooding) can increase migration even before a catastrophic disaster event occurs, through discourses of risk and interaction with other migration drivers. We look specifically at the interactions between discourses of risk and infrastructure decisions and argue that when climate change risks are identified, communities can suffer increasing neglect by development agencies and governing institutions. We investigate the role of circular, or labor-driven, migration in these communities and examine local insistence that rural villages and communities be maintained—even as community members relocate to more urban environments for work.

We draw comparisons between these two communities for multiple reasons. Both communities have been identified in the literature (Mortreux and Barnett 2009; Paton and Fairbairn-Dunlop 2010) and in the popular press (Chambers and Chambers 2007; Farbotko 2005; Mason et al. 2012; Pilkey and Young 2009) as being among the first "victims" of climate change (Farbotko and Lazrus 2012). In both cases, rising sea levels, significant erosion, and an increased intensity of storms have amplified the frequency and effects of flooding events—prompting disasters. In both Shishmaref and Nanumea, significant ecological changes collide with colonial histories and limited economic opportunities, producing an increased risk of major, life-threatening disasters. This risk, in turn, prompts discussion about migration as a long-term solution.

Comparing these communities is worthwhile given the extensive attention both have received as examples of the "face" of climate change and climate change-driven migration, the extreme extant and emerging ecological and social risks in the communities, and the similar patterns of colonial and post-colonial interactions between the communities and centers of power. Additionally, this chapter is one result of a nearly decade-long conversation between the two authors. Early anthropological efforts at climate change research were populated by a handful of graduate students, former ecologists, and (then rare) disaster anthropologists, who filled one or two panels at the American Anthropological Association and the Society for Applied Anthropology annual meetings in the early 2000s. It was during one of these panels that we first began comparing notes on Shishmaref and Tuvalu. We found there was significant basis for comparison then, and we continue to see links—both in the ecological circumstances that the communities face and in the way they have since become perceived and discussed by far-removed actors. Shishmaref is our primary case study in this chapter, with similarities and differences drawn to Nanumea to allow us deeper insights into our driving questions and to allow for both particular and more generalizable conclusions.

Methodology

Our case study comparison is based on many months of fieldwork and ongoing conversations with residents of the case study communities and other stakeholders who work on adaptive strategies for responding to climate impacts, including flooding events. In Shishmaref, Elizabeth Marino conducted more than sixty semi-structured interviews and twenty household surveys across a series of research projects between the years 2005 and 2010, including six months of concentrated fieldwork between 2008 and 2010. In addition to interviews, Marino carried out participant observation in the community both in daily life and, importantly, during meetings with federal, state, and local governing bodies to discuss options for relocation, migration, disaster mitigation, and erosion and flooding protection.

Heather Lazrus conducted twelve months of fieldwork in 2006 and 2007 in Tuvalu, primarily on Nanumea. Fieldwork included archival research, participant observation, and numerous conversations over this time period as well as fifty-six semi-structured interviews with Nanumean community leaders and other community members and one hundred household surveys. Interviews ranged from thirty minutes to more than two hours and were conducted in English and Tuvaluan with the aid of a translator, as appropriate.

Shishmaref, Alaska, and Nanumea, Tuvalu: Case Studies of Environmental Migration

Shishmaref, Alaska, and Nanumea, Tuvalu are situated in very different geographical, political, and social contexts, and yet both places are rural island communities experiencing the impacts of global climate change and are threatened with the possibility of catastrophic risk and displacement. Shishmaref, Alaska, is an Iñupiat community in western, coastal Alaska that sits on Sarichef Island off the coast of the Seward Peninsula between the Shishmaref Inlet and the Chukchi Sea. The village has a population of 563 (United States Department of Commerce 2010) and can only be reached by boat or plane. Today, the Kigiqtaamiut (Iñupiaq term meaning people of the island) harvest and consume an extensive variety of local subsistence foods. The economy in Shishmaref is a mixture of cash and subsistence, with a significant amount of trading and transfer happening across markets for access to traditional foods and commodities such as gas and ammunition, among other things. In Shishmaref, subsistence harvesting and the seasonal round still dominates annual cycles of travel, celebration, and lifestyle. Market employment on the island, however, is limited outside of medical, education, and government employment. The average income per capita in 2010 was US$10,203; 27 percent of residents live below the poverty line (AK DCCED 2014).

Nanumea is the northernmost atoll of Tuvalu, a low-lying Pacific Island country. The population of Tuvalu, approximately 10,000 people, is Polynesian and inhabits nine islands and atolls arcing across the Pacific Ocean between the latitude of 5° to 10° south and longitude of 176° to 180°. As a member of the United Nations, Tuvalu is active with the Association of Small Island States, a consortium of island and coastal states that continue to push for climate mitigation and adaptation assistance from the international community (Heileman 1993). Tuvalu is also a UN-designated "least developed country."

Similar to Shishmaref, Nanumea is home to approximately 600 people. It is accessible only by boat, and supplies and travelers are transported by an inter-island vessel that visits the outer islands once or twice a month. Nanumeans thrive on a mixed cash and subsistence economy, dominated by fishing, taro farming, and pig farming. Despite their remote location, contemporary Nanumean culture is strongly influenced by colonial and post-colonial forces; most of the population is Christian, and people on Nanumea enjoy access to electricity, Internet, and education up to secondary school. Yet, Nanumean culture also remains distinct, even from the other Tuvaluan island communities (Chambers and Chambers 2001; Stratford, Farbotko, and Lazrus 2013; Lazrus 2015).

Both Shishmaref and Nanumea exemplify places in the world where one manifestation of climate change is coastal flooding. This flooding, paired with changing social circumstances (Barnett and O'Neill 2010; Marino and Ribot 2012), could cause death and injuries to people and damage to housing and other essential infrastructure (IPCC 2012).

In Shishmaref and across the Arctic, increased erosion (USGAO 2003, 2009), increased storm activity (Hinzman et al 2005), and increased windiness (Huntington 2000), all linked to anthropogenic climate change, work in tandem to create flooding conditions. Six state-declared disasters have occurred since 1988 (Kinsman, DeRaps, and Smith 2013), and large storms can also cause rapid erosion. A fall storm in 2012 took up to thirty feet of land in a single night, which is significant for an island that is only three miles long and a half-mile wide. This erosion can be surprisingly quick, even for residents who have considerable experience in the region and with the extreme weather of the Alaskan coast, as exemplified in the following interview with Jennifer Demur, a resident who witnessed a number of the state flooding disasters.

> JD: That was pretty scary. Thinking how we're going to get out of here. You know, and is it really going to flood all the way over. But there was a lot of really excited people, and we were on the edge of the beach watching the waves and making sure nothing was going in. And I think that's when those houses were falling in. And I remember we were out there watching.
>
> EM: What were those people who owned those houses doing?
>
> JD: Rushing, emptying the house. There was lots of people helping.
>
> EM: Did you think those houses were in danger before the flood, or was it a surprise?
>
> JD: Well, we didn't think it would go that quick. (Interview with Jennifer Demur,[1] 23 September 2009)

These floods have resulted in extensive damage to infrastructure. According to Tony Weyiouanna, a relocation advocate from Shishmaref and former President of the Shishmaref Native Corporation, twenty-two houses have had to be moved away from the shoreline during and following large storms. So far no one has been severely injured or killed in these disaster events—but this is a significant fear among residents and stakeholders (Marino 2012). In 2006, the United States Army Corps of Engineers (USACE 2006) estimated that the island had up to fifteen years before continued erosion and flooding rendered the village uninhabitable (USACE 2006). Sea walls, revetment projects, and other erosion protection measures have been built to protect the island in the past and today, but these revetment projects have a limited lifespan. Nearly all stakeholders agree that relocation/migration is the only permanent solution for Shishmaref.

As in Shishmaref, communities in Tuvalu are starting to experience climate change impacts. Low-lying Pacific Islands face several challenges from climate change, including sea level rise that influences coastal hydrology and salt water incursion into freshwater supplies. Higher sea levels increase flooding from high tides and storm surge. Ocean acidification and increased sea surface temperatures damage marine ecosystems, disrupting coral colonies and removing the natural barriers they provide against storm surge from storms that may become more intense. Shifting precipitation patterns mean that less freshwater is available for drinking and household supplies (Nurse et al. 2014).

Similarly to the Alaska coast, Tuvalu experiences challenges with coastal erosion. While sea walls intended to prevent erosion have been constructed in some areas—often by international development organizations seeking to leave tangible evidence of their investments—they are often not effective and may actually serve to exacerbate erosion by channeling more wave energy onto the coast. On Nanumea, people living at one of the tips of the atoll, at the northern edge of the town, say that the ocean has been *kai fenua* (literally, eating the island) and can measure several yards of erosion that have occurred over the past four decades. Although Tuvalu lies slightly outside of the "cyclone belt" in which most cyclone activity in the South Pacific Ocean generally occurs, it has been significantly impacted by storms, which also affect the coastlines.

Surge from Cyclone Pam most recently hit Nanumea on 12 March 2015. Water swept across the atoll, carrying with it topsoil, graves, and material belongings. As the waves retreated, Nanumeans observed the new contours of their coastlines and the loss of land under some structures such as the Sunday school building.

No House, No Water—No Home? How Infrastructure Decisions Push Migration before the Big Floods Come

Apart from the risks of flooding, coastal erosion, and storm surges, discourses of risk and disaster create their own critical outcomes in both communities. In this section, we discuss the impacts of identifying risks in Shishmaref and Nanumea and how discourses of risk affect extra-local decisions about development and infrastructure improvements in the communities.

Shishmaref community members voted in 2002 to relocate off of the island to a more secure location on the mainland as a response to the threat of flooding and erosion. Interview data demonstrates that at the time, community members believed that a show of collective solidarity about moving would speed up the relocation process. This move never came to fruition, and today no infrastructure has been built in a new site on the mainland. For all intents and purposes, relocation in Shishmaref has not progressed significantly in the last decade.

What the vote unfortunately accomplished, however, was a nearly complete cessation of state or federal development money coming into the village. While most of the villages in the region have since received development in the form of new medical clinics, new housing, piped water systems, and/or a multipurpose building/cultural center, Shishmaref has received nearly none of this investment—linked to the lack of certainty about the future of the community.

In Shishmaref, public acknowledgement of risk has, therefore, created serious consequences for people choosing to stay in the village—such as the lack of a modern sanitation system and the associated health consequences and infectious disease rates that accompany the lack of piped water (Eichelberger 2010; Hennessy et al. 2008). Interview data demonstrate that residents attribute the negative health outcomes in the village to a lack of modern sanitation systems. Discourses of flooding risk and climate change, in some real sense, become embodied, therefore, as infectious diseases. Public acknowledgement of risk, in this case, lead to a cessation of development, which in turn encourages migration. Another outcome of the vote was the lack of funding and/or loan programs for new housing. The lack of housing is particularly problematic for young adults. Young adults returning from college or work elsewhere in the state are almost always required to move in with their parents in order to live in Shishmaref. Houses often have three and four generations—up to ten people—living in two-, three-, or four-bedroom homes. While multigenerational homes are common in rural Alaska, this extreme lack of housing is considered challenging and far from ideal—a situation that is becoming all the more problematic as the next generation has children:

> Even for people that do have housing, they have extended families living in them. . . . And then we've got a lot of nieces and nephews that are always over. And our neighbors are family still. With a smaller house, with everyone having more and more kids, each house gets smaller and smaller. (Interview with Bryce Eningowuk, 2008)

When an educated, returning young adult with employment can afford his or her own house, there is simply no infrastructure development for him or her to move into. This situation creates limited options for the millennial generation to remain in the village, particularly educated millennials who have plenty of opportunity to be independent elsewhere in Alaska (or beyond) and in other places that have running water.

In the above examples, climate change discourses isolate the village from critical modern infrastructure. This isolation from development creates its own push and pull factors for migration decisions, particularly those of young adults. In all of the interviews from Shishmaref, no one mentioned a family member that had moved because of flooding, but nearly everyone had a family member who could not find adequate housing.

As on Shishmaref, alongside severe ecological risks, people on Nanumea face challenges from inadequate infrastructure to maintain habitation of the atoll. Changing precipitation patterns and more frequent periods of drought threaten water security and may ultimately present a more proximate challenge to habitation than sea level rise and coastal flooding. Nanumea receives about 2,700 mm of rain per year (Sharp and Henson 1997), but actual water availability is limited by the technologies available to harvest rain water. Because much of the actual precipitation is lost through high evaporation and high soil porosity and permeability, the islands of the Tuvaluan archipelago are characterized scientifically as dry islands (McLean et al. 1991).

The infrastructure needed to ensure adequate water supplies on Nanumea is complex. All water supplies are collected from rooftops during rain events since the thin freshwater lens is brackish and not suitable for drinking water. With the construction of the first communal cement rainwater catchment cisterns in the early decades of the 1900s, Nanumeans no longer had to rely exclusively on the freshwater lens (Chambers 1984). While the government continues to maintain some larger cisterns, the main source of water for households is household rainwater catchment tanks. Most houses on Nanumea have an adjacent water tank. Rainwater can only be collected from the corrugated iron roofs that have largely replaced palm frond roofs for this reason and also contribute to the growing popularity of Western-style houses. Water must be collected near the point of use or transported manually, as there are no water or sewer pipes. During droughts, the water from household and community catchment tanks is rationed, but the cisterns and tanks run dry during extended periods without rain. Because changing precipitation patterns are likely to produce more intense but less frequent rain (Mimura et al. 2007), the storage capacity on the islands is not adequate to cope with this increasing variability. Unforeseen events, including funerals that bring large families together and stress water supplies, multiply the ecological impacts (Lazrus 2012b).

At the time of fieldwork, most households relied on water tanks made from ferro-cement, a material that requires maintenance and generally has a twenty-five-year life expectancy. The majority of these tanks had been installed in the 1980s by Save the Children and in the 1990s by the United Nations Development Program and were thus nearing the end of their expected life span. As Nanumea does not have the financial resources to supply new water tanks when old ones break or when new houses are constructed, the question arose about which development agency would invest in water infrastructure for an island that is slated to become uninhabitable due to rising seas. In a complex interplay, compounding factors increase the urgency of enhancing Nanumea's water supply to support continued inhabitation of the atoll:

the catchment systems are nearing the end of their anticipated life expectancy, the socially driven needs for water are increasing, and the local effects of climate change are intensifying (Lazrus 2012b)—but discourses that present Tuvalu and Nanumea as increasingly uninhabitable due to climate change may remove the availability of outside development dollars and aid (Lazrus 2015).

In both Shishmaref and Nanumea, we see that climate change creates significant impacts on coastal communities. What residents and researchers fear is that sea level rising, increased erosion, larger storm patterns, and flooding may culminate in a disaster scenario resulting in significant loss of life and the forceful and immediate evacuation and permanent displacement of residents. This scenario, however, is not the only climate-change related migration driver in either location. In both cases, discourses of risk and the nexus of infrastructure development and removal of funding streams also create risks and contribute to migration patterns and migration pressures outside of natural hazard scenarios. Moreover, the discourses of risk and resulting development decisions and lack of infrastructure investments are situated in complex histories of colonial governance. Thus, the dependence on external resources for local improvements perpetuates systemic vulnerabilities in the communities. In both Shishmaref and Nanumea, discourse about impending climate risk have served to undermine investment in local infrastructure—particularly water systems. Without the investments, infrastructure is increasingly inadequate and fails to maintain community needs regardless of the climate challenges the communities face. As a result, the choices for families and individuals to remain at home are compromised and can motivate decisions to relocate outside of disastrous events.

The Critical Difference between Circular Migration and Settlement Closure: Resisting Urbanization as an Adaptation Strategy for Climate Change Disasters

As may be expected, in Shishmaref and Nanumea, people migrate for many reasons including to further their education; to follow a job, a friend, a parent or child; and for the health services that exist in larger metropolitan areas. People are on the move—sometimes permanently, sometimes temporarily, and often frequently. These out-migration patterns, however, are identified locally as being critically distinct from village abandonment or settlement closure. Settlement closure before, or in the aftermath, of a large disaster event is a persistent fear of residents in Shishmaref and for good reason. In Alaska, the Army Corps of Engineers investigated the possibility of relocating residents to more urban environments as recently as 2005 (Schweitzer and Marino 2005). Here, we point to ways residents of Shishmaref and Nanumea may encourage and support the out-migration of individuals for education or labor reasons, among others, and yet insist on the maintenance of rural villages or the recreation of rural spaces in responses to climate change impacts. In these cases, climate change adaptation demands the possibility of recreating distinct human-ecological relationships, which may not be available in the same spaces people go to seek jobs or an education.

Demographic research in Alaska shows that a lack of jobs, not climate change, is the most significant cause of out-migration in rural Alaska (Huskey, Bermen, and Hill 2004). Unemployment rates in Shishmaref are likewise high. According to the American Community Survey, approximately 45.5 percent of workers in Shishmaref are out of the labor force (AK DCCED 2014), and the disparity between high unemployment rates in the village and the lower unemployment rates in larger hub areas create important incentives to relocate to more urban environments. Overall trends show that more people are moving out of rural Alaska than moving into rural Alaska (Huskey et al. 2004), and this trend has been consistent over time. In spite of these overall patterns of movement, return migration into the villages, and in-migration to rural spaces, is larger than economists and demographers might expect given the employment disparity. This creates what Lee Huskey, Matthew Berman, and Alexandra Hill call "Alaska's version of Todaro paradox" (2004: 79), a theory that rests on the fact that employment rates alone cannot explain migration decisions, particularly among Alaska Native populations within Alaska.

While overall rates of migration indicate that out-migration is dominant in rural Alaska, residents of Shishmaref have been adamant that permanent displacement outside of traditional subsistence territory is not an option for the community. Data collected through interviews found that 100 percent of fifty-four households interviewed did not want to relocate to the regional hubs of Nome or Kotzebue, Alaska, or to the larger metropolitan areas of Fairbanks or Anchorage (Schweitzer and Marino 2005). Removal or relocation to these larger urban areas was identified in interviews as creating Shishmaref "refugees" (interview with Richard Kuzuguk, 2009)—a population completely displaced. The banner on the Shishmaref Erosion and Relocation Coalition website reads: "We are worth saving" and claims that removal from subsistence territory is essentially the eradication of the Kigiqtaamiut culture. All relocation sites identified by Shishmaref residents are located within traditional subsistence territory, within which human-ecological relationships can be carried out in familiar and habitual ways.

In some cases, interviewees adamantly insisted that relocation in response to climate pressures to Nome, Kotzebue, or larger cities was not an option; yet, in years subsequent to initial interviews, these same friends and residents relocated to a larger, more urban area often for work. How can we explain this discrepancy?

One important aspect to contemporary life in rural Alaska, which we also see in Tuvalu, are the migration acts of moving back and forth between urban and rural spaces over the course of a year and/or over the course of a lifetime through both physical movement and through engaging in social ties with people from home. These migrations mimic international patterns of labor-driven, circular migration (Newland 2009; Skeldon 2012; Vertovec 2007); but the Shishmaref case also demonstrates unique qualities, including going home to get well, to combat alcoholism (Schweitzer and Marino 2005), to help with hunting, and to "breathe fresh air," which are not always tied to labor opportunities. These practices often characterize the lived distinction between "urban" and "rural" spaces and demarcate human-ecological relationships inherent in being home versus being away from home. This back-and-forth migration pattern supports the flow of goods, cultural values, and ideas. Migrants actively participate in social life in Shishmaref by returning for subsistence harvests, hunts, local celebrations, or times of trial, and by trading food and other goods from home across vast spaces and informal markets (Fienup-Riordan et al. 2000; Fogel-Chance 1993). These acts of social and cultural flexibility and fluidity between spaces, we argue, only work if there is a Shishmaref to which one can return and with which one can interact.

Interview data from Shishmaref are remarkably consistent in this area. Maintaining a village in traditional subsistence territory is a non-negotiable characteristic of any relocation plan. So, while out-migration is certain to occur and is encouraged by some community members, both individual interviews and the formal opinion of village leadership is absolutely resolute that Shishmaref must be maintained as a discrete, rural village in and around traditional subsistence territory.

Similar to the population of Shishmaref, many Nanumeans work overseas as seafarers on international vessels, teachers, and other vocations on the capital of Funafuti or beyond, in economic centers in Fiji, Australia, or New Zealand—where the Tuvaluan population is one of the fastest growing Pacific Islander groups according to the 2006 New Zealand Census. The important remittances that are sent back to family on Nanumea for family expenses mean that people who are working off-island are fully participating in social life at home (Farbotko and Lazrus 2012). Immigration programs, such as the Pacific Access Category, which allows seventy-five Tuvaluans per year to relocate to New Zealand, combined with work placement programs, help many Tuvaluans become New Zealand residents (Bedford and Bedford 2010). While not designed to address climate change, such programs may indirectly alleviate pressures in Tuvalu that arise from climate-induced environmental changes such as loss of land and reduced availability of water resources. Nanumeans usually spend some time off- island to pursue their education at one of the two secondary schools in the country located on different islands and for tertiary education at the Funafuti campus of the University of the South Pacific or overseas.

In addition to supporting social life at home, Nanumeans living off-island maintain strong Nanumean identities and connections to their home island. On Funafuti and in Wellington, New Zealand, the Nanumean communities proudly observe Nanumean customs and practices, including holidays that are unique to the home island, and maintain social relationships and family lineages from Nanumea. As among Shishmaref community members, Nanumeans in Nanumea, Funafuti, and Wellington agreed in interviews that even in the context of a highly mobile population, and in this case one that frequently crosses national borders, the ability to return home to Nanumea—whether or not that ability was ever actualized—was of paramount importance and is demonstrated through the flow of people, goods, and ideas that continually cross the water back and forth from Nanumea. In Tuvalu, the international mobility of a large segment of the population raises additional issues concerning citizenship and national identity, factors that also significantly constrain migration decisions (Farbotko, Stratford, and Lazrus 2015).

In both Shishmaref and Nanumea, the complexity of individuals' and families' movements reflects the numerous considerations and constraints present in contemporary migration decisions, which include economic, education, and health considerations but more often than not are also underscored by deep senses of home and belonging. The shifts that occur as people move across space and between rural and urban settings are also changes in the human-ecological relationships that characterize people's lives. Returning "home" allows human-ecological relationships to be maintained. The differences between temporary, or circular migration, and permanent relocation due to settlement closure or inadequate infrastructure are thus much more than demographic. Settlement closure would serve to turn otherwise temporary migration into permanent displacements, fundamentally shifting people's sense of home and belonging. In Shishmaref, this is demonstrated by community members' unanimous desire to remain a discrete, rural village, while among Nanumeans, it is evidenced in the ways people maintain ties to home even when living abroad. Research in Alaska has demonstrated that proximity to cultural peers is also a profound organizing force for maintaining minority cultures during periods of change and following eras of colonization and cultural genocide (Kingston and Marino 2010).

Conclusions

What we see in Shishmaref and Tuvalu is a complex mixture of ecological and social pressures that drive migration decisions through layered experiences of risk. In both communities, significant ecological changes increase the likelihood of a flooding disaster that could cause loss of life, livelihoods, critical infrastructure, and might ultimately force communities to relocate. However, in both communities these ecological changes interact with and are iteratively created by other risks such as the deterioration of infrastructure, discourses of climate change, and pressures to relocate outside of traditional subsistence territory.

In both cases, infrastructure decisions that occur in the context of climate change discourses can compromise contemporary livability of the islands—even before a major flooding event. In Tuvalu and Shishmaref, the identification as "victims" of climate change triggers the withdrawal of infrastructure investment by government and non-governmental agencies. The effect of infrastructure withdrawal is that even before ecological conditions render places uninhabitable, development decisions could challenge adequate living conditions in areas marked as "high risk."

We also find in both cases that migration is not a unidirectional decision. We see strong evidence that back-and-forth migrations are critical to maintaining cultural identity in Shishmaref and Tuvalu and even national identity in the case of Tuvalu. The implication of this for disaster and climate change scenarios is that while developers and disaster planners may see leaving a place, a territory, or even a nation as a permanent decision, and subsequently view places as becoming less viable and urbanization as an adaptive choice, communities that maintain traditional rural practices are more flexible in their sense of place. When disasters threaten the viability of places to exist, there is still a sociocultural demand for rural practices to continue, and adaptation strategies need to be structured to encapsulate cultural congruency as well as safety.

In places such as Shishmaref and Tuvalu, it appears as though large-scale ecological changes might force the displacement of entire communities during or following a major disaster. The possible displacement that may stem from this catastrophic scenario, however, interacts with and creates other migration pressures (i.e., economic needs, development policy, and rural infrastructure deterioration). In our analysis, the dichotomy between forced displacement and voluntary migration is blurred. Instead of strict typologies of migrations, we see individuals making decisions under constrained inventories of possibility, which includes the threat of a major disaster, as well as more persistent pressures of dilapidating infrastructure and the lack of jobs and services. What we also see consistently is the desire to participate in home. Disaster mitigation strategists should take this central tenet of participating in home into account. Even in these vastly different locations, the unbinding of human-ecological practices will not be a successful response to flooding, no matter how far from high water a community is located.

Elizabeth Marino is associate professor of anthropology and sustainability at Oregon State University—Cascades. She is interested in the relationships among climate change, vulnerability, slow and rapid onset disasters, human migration, and sense of place. Her research focuses on how historically and socially constructed vulnerabilities interact with climate change and disasters—including disaster policy, biophysical outcomes of disasters and climate change, and disaster discourses. She is also interested in how people make sense and meaning out of changing environmental and social conditions; and how people interpret risk. Her book *Fierce Climate, Sacred Ground: An Ethnography of Climate Change* was released in 2015.

Heather Lazrus is a project scientist in the Mesoscale and Microscale Meteorology Laboratory at the National Center for Atmospheric Research in Boulder, Colorado. Heather is an environmental anthropologist and uses the anthropological toolkit to investigate cultural mechanisms through which weather and climate risks are perceived, experienced, and addressed. Heather focuses on the interface between extreme weather and climate change. Current and recent research projects examine public perceptions of and behavior regarding flash floods, hurricanes, and drought. Her work has been published in journals including the *Annual Review of Anthropology, Human Organization*; *Global Environmental Change*; *Weather, Climate, and Society*; the *Bulletin of the American Meteorological Society*, and edited volumes.

Acknowledgment

An earlier version of this chapter was published in *Human Organization* 74(4), 2015.

Note

1. The names given here are not pseudonyms as requested by interviewees during the informed consent process.

References

Alaska Department of Commerce, Community, and Economic Development (AK DCCED). 2014. "2014 Alaska Community Information." *Department of Commerce, Community, and Economic Development: Division of Community and Regional Affairs*, 4 July. https://www.commerce.alaska.gov/web/dcra/communityinformation.aspx

Barnett, Jon, and Saffron O'Neill. 2010. "Maladaptation." *Global Environmental Change* 20(2): 211–13.

Bedford, Richard, and Charlotte Bedford. 2010. "International Migration and Climate Change: A Post- Copenhagen Perspective on Options for Kiribati and Tuvalu." In *Climate Change and Migration—South Pacific Perspectives*, ed. Bruce Burson, 89–134. Wellington, New Zealand: Victoria University Press.

Birk, Thomas, and Kjeld Rasmussen. 2014. "Migration from Atolls as Climate Change Adaptation: Current Practices, Barriers, and Options in Solomon Islands." *Natural Resources Forum* 38(1): 1–13.

Black, Richard, Dominic Kniveton, and Kerstin Schmidt-Verkerk. 2011. "Migration and Climate Change: Towards an Integrated Assessment of Sensitivity." *Environment and Planning-Part A* 43(2): 431–50.

Bronen, Robin. 2009. "Forced Migration of Alaskan Indigenous Communities Due to Climate Change: Creating a Human Rights Response." In *Linking Environmental Change, Migration, and Social Vulnerability*, ed. Anthony Oliver-Smith and Xiaomeng Shen, 70–88. Bonn, Germany: United Nations University Institute for Environment and Human Security.

———. 2011. "Climate-Induced Community Relocations: Creating an Adaptive Governance Framework Based in Human Rights Doctrine." *New York University Review of Law and Social Change* 35(2): 357–407.

Button, Gregory. 2010. *Disaster Culture: Knowledge and Uncertainty in the Wake of Human and Environmental Catastrophe.* Walnut Creek, CA: Left Coast Press.

Chambers, Anne. 1984. *Atoll Economy: Social Change in Kiribati and Tuvalu, No. 6.* Nanumea. 2nd ed. Canberra: Australian National University, Development Studies Centre.

Chambers, Keith, and Anne Chambers. 2001. *Unity of Heart: Culture and Change in a Polynesian Atoll Society.* Prospect Heights, IL: Waveland Press, Inc.

———. 2007. "Five Takes on Climate and Cultural Change in Tuvalu." *The Contemporary Pacific* 19(1): 294–306.

Crate, Susan. 2011. "Climate and Culture: Anthropology in the Era of Contemporary Climate Change." *Annual Review of Anthropology* 40: 175–94.

Eichelberger, Laura Palen. 2010. "Living in Utility Scarcity: Energy and Water Insecurity in Northwest Alaska." *American Journal of Public Health* 100(6): 1010–18.

Farbotko, Carol. 2005. "Tuvalu and Climate Change: Constructions of Environmental Displacement in the Sydney Morning Herald." *Geografiska Annaler B* 87(4): 279–93.

Farbotko, Carol, and Heather Lazrus. 2012. "The First Climate Refugees? Contesting Global Narratives of Climate Change in Tuvalu." *Global Environmental Change-Human and Policy Dimensions* 22(2): 382–90.

Farbotko, Carol, Elaine Stratford, and Heather Lazrus. 2015. "Climate Migrants and New Identities? The Geopolitics of Embracing or Rejecting Mobility." *Social and Cultural Geography* 17(4): 533–52.

Fienup-Riordan, Ann, William Tyson, Paul John, Marie Meade, and John Active. 2000. *Hunting Tradition in a Changing World: Yup'ik Lives in Alaska Today*. New Brunswick, NJ: Rutgers University Press.

Fogel-Chance, Nancy. 1993. "Living in Both Worlds: 'Modernity' and 'Tradition' among North Slope Iñupiaq Women in Anchorage." *Arctic Anthropology* 30(1): 94–108.

Heileman, Leo. 1993. "The Alliance of Small Island States (AOSIS): A Mechanism for Coordinated Representation of Small Island States on Issues of Common Concern." *Ambio* 22(1): 55–56.

Hennessy, Thomas W., Troy Ritter, Robert C. Holman, Dana L. Bruden, Krista L. Yorita, Lisa Bulkow, James E. Cheek, Rosalyn J. Singleton, and Jeff Smith. 2008. "The Relationship between In-Home Water Service and the Risk of Respiratory Tract, Skin, and Gastrointestinal Tract Infections among Rural Alaska Natives." *Journal Information* 98(11): 2072–78.

Hinzman, Larry, Neil D. Bettez, W. Robert Bolton, F. Stuart Chapin, Mark B. Dyurgerov, Chris L. Fastie, Brad Griffith, Robert D. Hollister, Allen Hope, Henry P. Huntington, et al. 2005. "Evidence and Implications of Recent Climate Change in Northern Alaska and Other Arctic Regions." *Climatic Change* 72(3): 251–98.

Hunter, Lori. 2005. "Migration and Environmental Hazards." *Population and Environment* 26(4): 273–302.

Huntington, Henry P. 2000. "Native Observations Capture Impacts of Sea Ice Changes." *Witness the Arctic* 8(1): 1–2.

Huskey, Lee, Matthew Berman, and Alexandra Hill. 2004. "Leaving Home, Returning Home: Migration as a Labor Market Choice for Alaska Natives." *The Annals of Regional Science* 38(1): 75–92.

Intergovernmental Panel on Climate Change (IPCC). 1990. "Policymakers Summary of the Potential Impacts of Climate Change." Report from Working Group II to the Intergovernmental Panel on Climate Change, Australia.

———. 2012. "Managing the Risks of Extreme Events and Disasters to Advance Climate Change Adaptation." A Special Report of Working Groups I and II of the Intergovernmental Panel on Climate Change, ed. Christopher B. Field, Vicente Barros, Thomas F. Stocker, Qin Dahe, David Jon Dokken, Kristie L. Ebi, Michael D. Mastrandrea, Katharine J. Mach, Gian-Kasper Plattner, Simon K. Allen, et al. New York: Cambridge University Press.

International Organization on Migration (IOM). 2008. "Migration and Climate Change." Migration Research Series, no. 31. Geneva, Switzerland: International Organization on Migration.

———. 2011. "Climate Change, Environmental Degradation, and Migration." 29–30 March 2011. Retrieved 7 January 2022 from http://www.iom.int/jahia/webdav/shared/shared/mainsite/microsites/IDM/workshops/climate-change-2011/background_paper.pdf.

Kingston, Deanna Marie, and Elizabeth Marino. 2010 "Twice Removed: King Islanders' Experience of 'Community' through Two Relocations." *Human Organization* 69(2): 119–28.

Kinsman, Nicole, Meagan R. DeRaps, and Jacquelyn R. Smith. 2013. "Preliminary Evaluation of Coastal Geomorphology and Geohazards on 'Kigiqtam Iglua' an Island Northeast of Shishmaref, Alaska." Fairbanks: Alaska Department of Natural Resources, Division of Geological and Geophysical Surveys.

Lazrus, Heather. 2012a. "Sea Change: Island Communities and Climate Change." *Annual Review of Anthropology* 41: 285–301.

———. 2012b. "Climate Change, Water, and Development in Daily Life in Tuvalu." In *Water, Cultural Diversity, and Global Environmental Change Emerging Trends, Sustainable Futures?*, ed. B. Rose Johnston, 88–92. New York: UNESCO and Springer.

———. 2015. "Risk Perception and Climate Adaptation in Tuvalu: A Combined Cultural Theory and Traditional Knowledge Approach." *Human Organization* 74(1): 52–61.

Maldonado, Julie K., Christine Shearer, Robin Bronen, Kristina Peterson, and Heather Lazrus. 2013. "The Impact of Climate Change on Tribal Communities in the US: Displacement, Relocation, and Human Rights." *Climatic Change* 120(3): 601–14.

Marino, Elizabeth. 2012. "The Long History of Environmental Relocation: Assessing Vulnerability Construction and Obstacles to Successful Relocation in Shishmaref, Alaska." In *Adding Insult to Injury: Climate Change, Social Stratification, and the Inequities of Intervention*, ed. Elizabeth Marino and Jesse Ribot. *Global Environmental Change* 22(2): 374–81.

———. 2013. "Environmental Migration: The Future of Anthropology in Social Vulnerability, Disaster, and Discourse." In *Environmental Anthropology: Future Directions*, ed. Helen Kopnina and Eleanor Shoreman-Ouimet, 188–203. New York: Routledge.

Marino, Elizabeth, and Jesse Ribot. 2012. "Special Issue Introduction: Adding Insult to Injury: Climate Change and the Inequities of Climate Intervention." *Global Environmental Change* 22(2): 323–28.

Mason, Owen K., James W. Jordon, Leanne Lestak, and William F. Manley. 2012. "Narratives of Shoreline Erosion and Protection at Shishmaref, Alaska: The Anecdotal and the Analytical." In *Pitfalls of Shoreline Stabilization*, ed. J. Andrew Cooper and Orin Pilkey, 73–92. Amsterdam: Springer.

Massey, Douglas S., William G. Axinn, and Dirgha J. Ghimire. 2010. "Environmental Change and Out-Migration: Evidence from Nepal." *Population and Environment* 32(2–3): 109–36.

McLean, Roger F., Paul F. Holthus, Peter L. Hosking, and Colin D. Woodroffe. 1991. *Tuvalu Land Resources Survey: Nanumea.* Auckland, New Zealand: Department of Geography, University of Auckland.

Mimura, Nobuo, Leonard Nurse, Roger McLean, John Agard, Lino Briguglio, Penehuro Lefale, Rolph Payet, and Graham Sem. 2007. "Small Islands." In *Climate Change 2007: Impacts, Adaptation, and Vulnerability*, ed. Contribution of Working Group II to the Fourth Assessment Report of the Intergovernmental Panel on Climate Change, Martin L. Parry, Osvaldo F. Canziani, P. Jean Palutikof, Paul J. van der Linden, and Clair E. Hanson, 687–716. Cambridge: Cambridge University Press.

Mortreux, Colette, and Jon Barnett. 2009. "Climate Change, Migration, and Adaptation in Funafuti, Tuvalu." *Global Environmental Change* 19(1): 105–12.

Myers, Candice A., Tim Slack, and Joachim Singelmann. 2008. "Social Vulnerability and Migration in the Wake of Disaster: The Case of Hurricanes Katrina and Rita." *Population and Environment* 29(6): 271–91.

Myers, Norman. 1993. "Environmental Refugees in a Globally Warmed World." *Bioscience* 43(11): 752–61.

Newland, Kathleen. 2009. *Circular Migration and Human Development.* Research Paper 2009/42. New York: United Nations Development Programme.

Nurse, Leonard A., Roger F. McLean, John Agard, Lino P. Briguglio, Virginie Duvat-Magnan, Reiko Obokata, Luisa Veronis, and Robert McLeman. 2014. "Empirical Research on In-

ternational Environmental Migration: A Systematic Review." *Population and Environment* 36(1): 111–35.
Oliver-Smith, Anthony. 1996. "Anthropological Research on Hazards and Disasters." *Annual Review of Anthropology* 25: 303–28.
———. 2004. "Theorizing Vulnerability in a Globalized World: A Political Ecology Perspective." In *Mapping Vulnerability: Disasters, Development, and People*, ed. Greg Bankoff, George Frerks, and Dorothea Hillhorst, 10–24. London: Earthscan.
———. 2013. "Disaster Risk Reduction and Climate Change Adaptation: The View from Applied Anthropology." *Human Organization* 72(4): 275–82.
Paton, Kathryn, and Peggy Fairbairn-Dunlop. 2010. "Listening to Local Voices: Tuvaluans Respond to Climate Change." *Local Environment* 15(7): 687–98.
Pilkey, Orrin H., and Rob Young. 2009. *The Rising Sea.* Seattle, WA: Island Press.
Schweitzer, Peter, and Elizabeth Marino. 2005. *Shishmaref Co-Location Cultural Impact Assessment.* Seattle, WA: Tetra Tech Inc.
Sharp, Roslyn, and Barbara Henson, eds. *1997 National Environmental Management Strategy.* Apia, Samoa: South Pacific Regional Environment Programme.
Skeldon, Ronald. 2012. "Going Round in Circles: Circular Migration, Poverty Alleviation, and Marginality." *International Migration* 50(3): 43–60.
Smit, Barry, and Johanna Wandel. 2006. "Adaptation, Adaptive Capacity, and Vulnerability." *Global Environmental Change* 16(3): 282–92.
Stratford, Elaine, Carol Farbotko, and Heather Lazrus. 2013. "Tuvalu, Sovereignty and Climate Change: Considering Fenua, the Archipelago and Emigration." *Island Studies Journal* 8(1): 67–83.
United States Army Corps of Engineers (USACE). 2006. *Village Erosion Technical Assistance Program: An Examination of Erosion Issues in the Communities of Bethel, Dillingham, Kaktovik, Kivalina, Newtok, Shishmaref, and Unalakleet.* Washington, DC: United States Army Corps of Engineers.
United States General Accounting Office (USGAO). 2003. "Alaska Native Villages: Most Are Affected by Flooding and Erosion, but Few Qualify for Federal Assistance." Retrieved 17 September 2014 from http://www.gao.gov/new.items/d04142.pdf.
United States General Accounting Office (USGAO). 2009. "Alaska Native Villages: Limited Progress Has Been Made on Relocating Villages Threatened by Flooding and Erosion." Retrieved 17 September 2014 from http://www.gao.gov/new.items/d09551.pdf.
United States Department of Commerce. 2012. "Alaska: 2010, Population and Housing Unit Counts." *United States Census 2010*, June 2012. Retrieved 2 September 2015 from https://www.census.gov/prod/cen2010/cph-2-3.pdf.
Vertovec, Steven. 2007. *Circular Migration: The Way Forward in Global Policy?* COMPAS Working Paper 4. Oxford: International Migration Institute, University of Oxford.
Warner, Koko. 2010. "Global Environmental Change and Migration: Governance Challenges." *Global Environmental Change* 20(3): 402–13.

PART II

Challenging the Borders of Care

The intersections between migration and health care provision can often be fraught for populations, patients, kin, and practitioners alike. While true of all healing systems, this complexity is particularly true of biomedical care, which, with its roots in Western hegemony and its increasing intersections with neoliberal agendas, is often not set up to support the health of people on the move. Biomedicine has been shown to enforce political, economic, and social norms that help govern human bodies. Such power relations are not experienced equally, and migrants are often especially at risk for substandard, insufficient, or coercive care. At the same time, some health institutions and practitioners work on the forefront of challenging these inequities in access and quality of care. The ethnographic work in these chapters takes us into three very different efforts to do exactly this.

This section asks:

How do migration and migrants challenge the borders of biomedical care? Alternatively, how have migrants negotiated these borders, and how have biomedical practitioners adapted? How does this impact the practice of biomedicine in different contexts?

Chapter 4 documents how, along with migrants, alternative modalities of healing and suffering travel, challenging local, homogeneous clinical contexts and norms. The chapter illustrates how, in certain conditions, clinicians are able to offset the traditional disciplinary borders of their practice, making space for clinical innovations that better address migrant patients' experiences and needs. By doing so, clinicians also challenge the unequal dynamic between hegemonic and subaltern cultures that are often reproduced in the context of healthcare.

Beyond challenging the epistemic borders of biomedical practice, migration and migrants shine a light onto the social dimensions of illness that typically elude traditional health institutions. Chapter 5 documents how, in the context of chronic illness, migrant patients' structural vulnerability calls for the intervention and collaboration of professionals from different categories—both those outside the medical realm and those operating at the community level.

Finally, chapter 6 looks at challenges to biomedical (and political) hegemony from an original perspective: migrant doctors returning to provide humanitarian aid in their own countries of origin. These migrant doctors' engagement unsettles the figure of white American or European global aid workers that often dominate the literature and the media. It also disrupts the traditional East-West and North-South border divides that ordinarily define the context of humanitarian aid and lead to hierarchies of humanitarians and hierarchies of care.

4

Translating Fanon in the Italian Context
Rethinking the Ethics of Treatment in Psychiatry

Cristiana Giordano

Culture is conflict.
—Psychologist, Centro Franz Fanon

The mental health of immigrants in most European countries and in North America raises unresolved questions about psychiatry, a discipline that remains a critical frame for exploring legacies of colonial violence and postcolonial transition (Keller 2007). In Italy, ethnopsychiatry and its objects of inquiry offer privileged windows into the experience of migration of postcolonial populations and its effects on the ethics and politics of therapeutic treatment. In this chapter, I examine the position of a group of Italian ethnopsychiatrists on the use of culture in the therapeutic setting. My reflections are based on two years of ethnographic fieldwork at the Centro Franz Fanon, a clinic in Northern Italy that offers psychological support to immigrants, refugees, torture victims, as well as to Italian social workers, religious people, and volunteers who work with them. My aim here is twofold: (1) to situate the clinical practice of this group of practitioners within the larger landscape of Italian psychiatry and medical anthropology, and within theories of domination and culture developed by Frantz Fanon and Tobie Nathan; (2) to reflect upon ethnopsychiatry as a contested field that raises a series of complex questions about migration, mental health, and identity, and thus opens up the possibility to rethink clinical work as a political space, for both foreign and Italian patients alike.

Ethnopsychiatry's legacy has been traced back to the works of colonial doctors such as John Colin Carothers and Octave Mannoni (Beneduce and Martelli 2005; Beneduce 2005), and in Italy to the experience of community-based psychiatry, Antonio Gramsci's political thought, and Ernesto de Martino's anthropological research (Pandolfi and Bibeau 2005). I follow a similar historical and textual trajectory, and also turn to authors who have addressed the colonial and post-colonial implications of psychiatric interventions both in Europe and in former colonies. By creating a conversation between texts and passages of interviews with ethno-psychiatrists, I elucidate their clinical use of culture, and situate the political dimension of this kind of clinical work within larger debates on mental health and difference. While showing the importance of ethnopsychiatry's interventions, I also point to the implications of using cultural material in the therapeutic setting and the risks of failing to subject psychiatric categories to a real critique when the focus of therapeutic work is exclusively "the other."

In Italy, access to health care is a legal right of citizens and non-citizens alike. Despite this fact, there remains a significant disparity in access to services. In the text of the National Health Plan (2002–2004) the Department of Health denounces what it describes as "a substantial lack of flexibility in the offering of services in the face of the new health problems of these new groups of clients" (Beneduce and Martelli 2005). After the closure of the mental hospital, psychiatric services in Italy have been increasingly community-based in an attempt to limit the risks of medicalization and the stigmatization of mental illness. Nevertheless, in practice, access to mental health care has often been off-limits for migrants. As a result, alternative spaces of psychological and psychiatric care—such as the Centro Fanon—have been designed for foreigners. These independent initiatives have received public funding without, however, being recognized in their own right as part of the public health system.[1] They remain marginal to the domain of public policy and stand as a critique of the institutional structure of health care.

Clearly, ethnopsychiatry operates from its inception within the domain of political action. The recent debates on ethnopsychiatry in Europe show that speaking about culture in relation to suffering and therapy is a highly controversial topic, which risks generating accusations of racism (Fassin 2000; Nathan 2003; Beneduce 2007). Reasons for this tension and controversy can be found in the history of psychiatry (Beneduce 2008), but questions of culture and power relationships have re-emerged today despite the fact that ethnopsychiatry and transcultural psychiatry position themselves in opposition to colonial psychiatry.[2] On the one hand, culture is an increasingly politicized domain of public discourse, inasmuch as it is through the language of cultural difference that the relationship between immigrants and receiving countries is articulated; on the other hand, ethnopsychiatry, because it is committed to the treatment of foreigners finds itself within a highly politicized terrain in which questions of citizenship and borders, mental health and rights intersect in complex ways.

The Centro Frantz Fanon was established in 1996 by a group of psychiatrists, psychologists, anthropologists, and cultural mediators as a political response to the forms of discrimination foreigners faced in Italian public institutions. Part of a revival of clinical ethnopsychiatry in other European countries, this center is a site where, through the incorporation of different etiologies of mental suffering and healing approaches, a strong counter-discourse to normative psychiatry is produced. In the context of ethno-psychiatric treatment, the patient's cultural background provides therapists with a framework for a new practice of listening in which the patient's claims to the magic and the supernatural as constitutive orders of subjectivity are taken seriously and often used as therapeutic tools (Beneduce 1998).[3] What is at stake here is the question of difference in relationship to healing and suffering, and its potential to critique institutions and colonial experiences.[4]

Tobie Nathan's clinical experience in France has had an important impact on the Italian context.[5] While the Centro Fanon draws from Nathan's goal of reconnecting migrants to their culture of origin as a therapeutic technique, other philosophical and medical traditions—such as phenomenology, existentialism, the work of Ernesto de Martino, and Franco Basaglia's experience of *psichiatria democratica* (democratic psychiatry)—also influence the Centro's clinical approach. The specificity of Italian ethnopsychiatry can only be understood against the backdrop of the debates around the de-institutionalization of the mentally ill and the radical critique of public institutions initiated by Franco Basaglia, and the de-institutionalization movement in the early 1970s (Pandolfi and Bibeau 2005). Crucial to the Italian context is also the work of Antonio Gramsci and his reflection on the complex relationships between hegemony and subaltern cultures, and on the role of the organic intellectual in creating a field of political action that could involve the subalterns in the definition of what counts as politics. Moreover, Frantz Fanon's denunciation of colonial power relations and the violence embedded in institutions represents the theoretical ground on which the group of practitioners and cultural mediators base their reflections on discrimination and race and devise training for mental health practitioners and social workers who work in public services (Beneduce 2007).

Franco Basaglia: Psychiatry without *Manicomio*

> Interviewer: Doctor Basaglia, to conclude, are you more interested in the patient or in his illness?
>
> Basaglia: Definitely in the patient![6]

The recent revival of ethnopsychiatry in Italy has its roots in a long standing Italian intellectual critique of public institutions. Franco Basaglia embodies a tradition of politically engaged mental health reform originating in the 1960s and 1970s. Recognized as the leading figure of the democratic psychiatry movement in Europe, Basaglia (1924–1981) became the director of the Trieste mental asylum in 1971 where, together with a group of colleagues, nurses, and social workers, he started a systematic critique of mental health institutions and the violence embedded therein.

According to Basaglia, the solution to the closed and violent structure of the *manicomio*[7] was to be found not in humanitarian gestures that increased the degree of dependency between reformers and patients, but rather in questioning the power relationships that characterized the practice of institutional psychiatry. He interpreted mental illness as a sociopolitical problem and envisioned a public psychiatry able to comprehend suffering and social misery outside the hospital walls. Influenced by the work of Michel Foucault (1961) and Erving Goffman (1961) on the asylum, Basaglia offered a complex analysis of the interrelation between mental illness and society's response to the management of suffering. This critique set the foundation for a process of self-reflection on the part of mental health practitioners and led to the abolition of the mental hospital in Italy in 1978.

For Basaglia, the asylum was a microsocial architectural space that reproduced perversions in human relationships and created an illness specific to itself: institutional psychosis or institutionalism (Scheper-Hughes and Lovell 1987: 11). The institution foreclosed any possibility of listening to, and empathizing with the patient's life world:

> In order to truly face "illness," we should be able to encounter it *outside* of institutions. By this I mean, not only outside of the psychiatric institution, but *outside* of any other institution whose function is to label, codify, and fix those who belong to them into roles. Does there really exist an *outside* from where to take action before institutions destroy us? Can't we, instead, deduce that what we know of the "illness" appearance is always, anyway, its institutional appearance? (Basaglia 1968: 374, author's translation, italics in original)

By highlighting the institutional construction of mental illness as a "disease," Basaglia radically questioned psychiatrists' practice and their social responsibility vis-à-vis patients. Influenced by existentialism and the phenomenological approach to mental illness developed by Ludwig Binswanger and Eugène Minkowski, Basaglia's focus was to re-evaluate the encounter between doctor and patient that the asylum denied and made impossible due to its hierarchical and closed structure. To enter the life world of the mentally ill, one had to break free from the situation of oppression instituted by the asylum's apparatus of control. The diagnostic apparatus kept the psychiatrist from exploring what was behind symptoms and the expressions of suffering. Basaglia wrote: "we believe that in order to have a relationship with an individual, it is necessary to establish it independently of the label by which the person has been defined" (1968: 31, author's translation).

In my conversations with ethnopsychiatrists at the Centro Fanon, Basaglia's legacy was often evoked as central to the contemporary setting of their clinical interventions. Simona Taliani, a psychologist trained in ethnopsychiatry and medical anthropology, once explained to me:

> We provide a clinical space where we put diagnoses and psychodynamic interpretations aside in order to listen to what the other has to say about his/her malaise. . . . Our methodology is meant to accompany the person in exploring all the etiologies that they have in mind. . . . In this way, we are engaged in a political effort to see the other as a political subject that has something to say about their story and history.[8]

In line with Basaglia's teaching, diagnoses are seen as an expression of the hegemonic power of the institutions that foreclose a real therapeutic encounter.

For Basaglia, the phenomenological approach allowed psychiatrists to expose themselves directly to patients' life worlds. Empathy with the patient allows for the creation of "a terrain of encounter . . . which allows one to find a path from which to start a therapeutic relationship" (Basaglia 1981: 4, author's translation). As Simona Taliani put it, ethnopsychiatry positions the patient as a political subject "not because s/he is a victim of human trafficking or of torture, or an asylum seeker, but because they tell us about their suffering . . . by using their mother tongues and local etiologies." In the ethnopsychiatric setting the patient is in a position where power dynamics are for a moment inverted "because the most competent one is not the doctor but the patient herself." This therapeutic relationship allows for a different kind of empathy with the patient's symbolic and psychic life. As she put it: "the use of the mother tongue in therapy sessions is not because we are anthropologically sensitive to the patient's cultural difference, but because the mother tongue is a political instrument to say certain things."[9]

When the phenomenological analysis was no longer sufficient to explain the class nature of illness and the larger sociopolitical context that determined its modes of expression, Basaglia turned to Gramsci and other Italian Marxist thinkers. Understanding madness not as a mere social product as a positivist logic would explain it, but rather as a complex nexus of contradictions (institutional, ideological, ethical, medical, political, social) that find their expression in the bodies of patients, questioning the structure of medical knowledge itself, its practices and representations—all these goals allowed Basaglia to bring to the fore the issues relating to psychiatry and its relationship to the law.

The traditional asylums were still governed by the 1904 law that positioned psychiatry within the criminal justice system, assigning it the function of *custodia* (control, custody) rather than of *cura* (care). Basaglia was one of the main advocates of the 1978 Law 180 (*Legge Basaglia,* Basaglia's Law), which ratified the closure of the *manicomio*, prohibited building new asylums, and promoted the organization of a community-based psychiatry through mental health centers. By involving the community in changing cultural attitudes toward deviance, this law also changed the relationship between psychiatry and the legal system, and ended the exclusive management of mental illness by doctors. It confronted the old contradiction between *custodia* (control) and *cura* (treatment), and it redefined the institution as a positive space in which a different kind of encounter could take place.[10]

At the Centro Fanon, the political dimension of Italian community psychiatry intersected with the cultural approach of ethnopsychiatry. Roberto Beneduce once explained to me how the Centro came into existence and the motivations, both clinical and political, behind it:

> There was a desire on our part not to lose sight of the legacy of Italian community psychiatry. From our point of view, that legacy was not at odds with the opening up of the cultural area . . . . It wasn't easy to bring together

> the political and the cultural in the clinical work with immigrant patients because even the most sensitive Italian psychiatry never intentionally developed its medical anthropological intuitions.[11]

According to Beneduce, directing the critique to institutional settings prevents one from seeing how mental illness is constructed and reproduced not only inside the psychiatric institution, but also in the social imaginary. For him, focusing on the social dimension of suffering was the "undelivered promise of the writings of some psychiatrists and psychoanalysts between the [19]60s and [19]70s." An immigrant himself from the south to the north of Italy, Beneduce drew from both his personal and professional experience to translate Basaglia's legacy into a way to work with the immigrant population.

Basaglia's (1968) critique of the relationships of domination within institutions echoes Fanon's (1963) unveiling of the institutional roots of violence in the colonial context. However, Basaglia contrasted Fanon's work in the psychiatric hospital in Algeria with his own. It was in Algiers that Fanon clarified his position as a politicized psychiatrist by realizing that the doctor-patient relationship is always defined by the system. Since the "therapeutic act" is an "act of silent acceptance of the system," Fanon saw revolution as the only way to act against the institution. Basaglia wrote:

> Fanon was able to choose revolution. We, for objective reasons, are prevented from doing it. In our reality, we still need to continue to experience the contradictions of the system that over-determines us, by managing an institution that we deny, by performing a therapeutic act that we refuse, by preventing that the institution . . . continues to be *only* functional to the system. We attempt to resist the flattery of new scientific ideologies that tend to hide those contradictions, which it is our duty to make explicit. *We are aware of the absurdity of this wager: we want to keep values alive, while non-rights, inequality, and the quotidian death of man are turned into legislative principles.* (1968: 379–80, author's translation, italics in original).

Basaglia's idea was to work from within the conundrum of the system in order to address the contradictions of an institution that he fundamentally rejected. The constant process of undoing psychiatry from within differed from Fanon's engagement in the revolution. Basaglia called this project *l'utopia della realtà* (The utopia of reality, 2005). For Fanon, on the other hand, revolution required the radical rupture and negation of the mental institution by stepping outside of it, which he did by resigning from his position as a clinical psychiatrist in the hospital in Algiers.

Basaglia's vigilant critique of state institutions, coupled with the urge to reform public services in the domain of public health, still characterize Italian ethnopsychiatry. While this more politicized approach to illness and healing was at first oriented toward the economically and politically marginalized, since the early 1980s, ethnopsychiatry has increasingly addressed marginalization and domination through a specific focus on migrant communities. It argues that health care for migrants is a political issue rather than a strictly medical one. Basaglia's legacy shapes the political debates arising from the epistemological uncertainty that mainstream psychiatry is forced to confront in the treatment of migrants.

When Foucault (1994) wrote about the great reforms of psychiatric power and thought over the last century, he argued that they placed the power relations embedded in psychiatry at the center of the field and fundamentally questioned them. Great reforms are attempts to displace power, to unmask it, and nullify it. As Foucault observed: "The whole of modern psychiatry is fundamentally pervaded by antipsychiatry, if one understands by this everything that calls back into question the role of the psychiatrist formerly charged with producing the truth of illness in the hospital space" (1994: 45). Several antipsychiatries have traversed the history of modern psychiatry and contemporary Italian ethnopsychiatry is one of them.[12]

Ernesto de Martino's Cultural Apocalypse

Trained as a religious historian, and renowned as a philosopher and ethnographer, Ernesto de Martino engaged in a serious re-evaluation of the intersections of history, religion, psychoanalysis, psychiatry, anthropology, and political theory, and contributed to the questioning of Western diagnostic categories and apparatuses (Bartocci and Prince 1998; Beneduce and Martelli 2005). His reflections were influenced by phenomenology, Antonio Gramsci's Marxism, and Benedetto Croce's historicism. His work, in the 1940s, anticipated many of the epistemological concerns that lie at the heart of current ethnopsychiatry, including questions of mental health, diagnostic categories, and the conundrum of difference.

Ernesto de Martino pointed out the importance of political engagement on the part of the ethnographer in regard to his/her object of inquiry. Although his initial interest was in colonial contexts, he later shifted his ethnographic focus to the marginalized of his own society. His fieldwork in rural southern Italy continued a tradition of anthropology "at home" pursued by Italian researchers (Seppilli 2001). According to de Martino, certain magic-religious rituals and therapeutic techniques in Western societies were deeply linked to both hegemonic and subaltern logics of power and domination between different socio-economic classes. The ethnographer had the responsibility of illustrating these logics in all their complexity. De Martino focused on the study of rituals of possession and on their meanings for the individual and their relationships with society.

His first book, *Naturalismo e storicismo nell'etnologia* (Naturalism and historicism in ethnology, 1941) begins with a reflection on the crisis of Western civilization and a call for a critical analysis of the history of the West as a fundamental goal of ethnographic work. His philosophy was later referred to as *etnocentrismo critico* (critical ethnocentrism): our study of the other necessarily entails a critical analysis of our own analytical categories. In *La fine del mondo* (The end of the world), an unfinished manuscript published posthumously in 1977, de Martino returns to the project idea of the undoing of Western categories of analysis. By employing these categories in the study of the other, we will only see projections of ourselves in the alien; on the other hand, by not using them, nothing can be observed. To resolve this paradox, the Western ethnographer must be aware of the historical context that produced his analytical framework in as much as it is not pertinent to other cultures. Through this *epoché*, we contribute to anthropological knowledge (1977: 410).

When ethnopsychiatrists at the Centro Fanon refer to de Martino's work, they acknowledge the importance of this *epoché* that allows for the possibility of listening—within the space of the clinic—to the patients' different etiologies. The experience of migration often creates a limbo in which several explanations of symptoms are possible and appropriate. For instance, in the case of a Nigerian woman who was referred to the Centro by the public department of mental health where she had been diagnosed with schizophrenia, the ethnopsychiatric group suspended that diagnosis and asked her in what terms her symptoms would be described in Nigeria, by her family, villagers, and by her healer. In this therapeutic process, other etiologies used to understand her experience, including the language of possession and witchcraft, of devotion to Mami Wata, and different forms of ties associated to voodoo rituals were discussed.

As Piero Coppo (2005) points out, ethnopsychiatry is first of all a method that allows for different etiologies to be evoked and used in the clinical encounter. Ethnopsychiatry then is not a subfield of psychiatry but a way of reconceiving the clinical response to the patient. The encounter with alterity—be it ethnographic or psychopathological—asks for a radical revision of the disciplines that history has produced. Ethnopsychiatry looks at psychiatry as a historical product, a culturally shaped *savoir-faire* among others (Coppo 2005). This kind of revision resonates with de Martino's invitation to critique Western consciousness.

Throughout his work, de Martino was concerned with what he terms the *crisi della presenza* (crisis of presence) of modern civilization, which involves the place of the individual within society. The "crisis of presence" refers to the existential anxiety that one might be effaced by situations that challenge the individual's ability to handle external and internal realities. Influenced by Martin Heidegger, Jean-Paul Sartre, and Georg W. F. Hegel's master-slave dialectic, de Martino developed his own understanding of what it means to be in the world (Saunders 1993). In *Il mondo magico* (The magic world, [1948] 2000), de Martino first introduced the "crisis of presence" through a discussion of the Malaysian context. He described the experience of *latah*, the dissociative state in which a person becomes vulnerable to external influences, imitating and echoing others, and generally losing the boundaries of his/her own personality and sense of self (see Wazir 1990; Winzeler 1995; Simon 1996). In this crisis, "the distinction between presence [as consciousness] and the world that makes itself present crumbles" (de Martino [1948] 2000: 93). He refers to the subject's risk of no longer being in the world, of "not being there" ("il rischio di non esser-ci").

Although de Martino seems to be interested in the "crisis of presence" more from existential and historical perspectives than from a strictly psychoanalytical one, in an article entitled "Crisi della presenza e reintegrazione religiosa" (Crisis of presence and religious reintegration) published in the philosophical review *Aut Aut* in 1956, he establishes a parallel between certain instances of loss of presence and mental illness. The person suffering from a mental illness may lose their ability to engage dialectically with the world and to relate to the object as outside one's self. The subject loses their ability to relate to the world symbolically and instead identifies with it. At the core of this crisis is the anxiety that "underlines the threat of losing the distinction between subject and object, between thoughts and action, between representation and judgment, between vitality and morality: it is the cry of one who is wobbling on the edge of the abyss" (1956: 25).

De Martino assigns the function of resolving the crisis of presence to religious rituals which re-establish the ties between the individual and the social, and re-anchor the subject within the symbolic order through what he calls *il riscatto culturale* (cultural redemption). Religious and magical rituals help people overcome the sense of loss and alienation experienced within the crisis of presence by providing the subject with a structure that allows the re-establishment of boundaries between themselves and the world. Traditional and religious therapies aim at reintegrating the individual into the community. Idiosyncrasies are translated into the mythical narrative and in the structure offered by rituals (Beneduce and Martelli 2005: 376). In this sense, de Martino's reflections are a prelude to contemporary ethnopsychiatric practice, which figures religious rituals and the vocabulary of magic as therapeutic. Encouraging patients to perform rituals that are meaningful to them, as well as referring to the language of witchcraft and possession are among the therapeutic modalities that ethnopsychiatrists apply in their clinical work. These experiences are often described by clinicians at the Centro through the category of "culture" and are represented as therapeutic tools. As discussed in more depth later in this chapter, allowing for alternative modalities of healing and suffering within the ethnopsychiatric setting can have an ambivalent outcome: while creating an alternative space to public healthcare institutions, it also risks reifying magic-religious practices by confining them to the domain of "culture" as a static field that can be turned into another diagnostic category. While knowledge of cultural difference is important for clinicians, it is also crucial to let the individual's psyche find its own paths within and outside of the constraints imposed by culture (Rechtman 2000).

De Martino was in conversation with several Italian psychiatrists and psychoanalysts on the question of the crisis of presence and its pertinence to psychopathology and clinical work, including Giovanni Jervis (1994), Bruno Callieri (2001), and Michele Risso (Risso and Böker 1992). In de Martino's work, the crisis of presence figures as an existential category that produces anthropological understanding and addresses the broader question of the historicity of man. The crisis is linked to the question of *apocalissi culturali* (cultural apocalypses), which de Martino develops in *La fine del mondo*. Here de Martino reflects on the uncertain boundaries between the pathological (and individual) and cultural dimensions, between the psychological register and the historical-anthropological temporality of being. Mariella Pandolfi and Gilles Bibeau (2005) argue that de Martino's project is the first attempt in anthropological theory to reflect on these issues from multiple angles: on the one hand, he considers the macro-dimension of cultural apocalypses and, on the other hand, he is attentive to the micro-dimensions of the catastrophic event, or the risk of loss of self and pathology. An exterior catastrophic event can put the sense of self in danger but this crisis can also be translated into a return to the world in ways that were previously unimaginable. Nonetheless, subjectivity is inherently at risk of losing itself. It is precisely this dimension of risk, both ontological and historical, that for de Martino constitutes subjectivity.

In *La fine del mondo*, de Martino sketches the first critical analysis of psychological and psychiatric categories, thus anticipating recent medical-anthropological critiques of diagnostic criteria and their application within the context of Italian ethnopsychiatry. He argues that cultural psychiatry can illuminate the links between psychological disorders and the failure of culture's task of holding the individual and assigning meaning to events. Not only does a transcultural approach to psychiatry allow for a study of the sociocultural dimensions of mental disorders and the recognition of the effectiveness of traditional, culture-sensitive therapies, but it also contributes to critical epistemological approaches to the diagnostic categories of psychiatry as a whole. When ethno-psychiatrists at the Centro Fanon describe their process of assessing the patient's psychological condition, they refer to their "prudent use of psychiatric diagnoses," as one ethnopsychiatrist put it. The aim is to let psychiatric diagnoses be undone and questioned by the patient's own metaphors, interpretations, and worldview (Kirmayer 1999). In this way, multiple models are at play and provide different angles on symptoms and experiences, without reproducing the hegemonic discourse on mental health.

Colonial and Postcolonial Disorders

Categories of psychiatry and medicine played a decisive role in the confrontation between dominant and dominated cultures, even when they aimed at fostering cultural sensitivity. In the name of respect and sensitivity for difference, old power dynamics can reemerge under different disguise. For example, the ethnopsychiatrists I interviewed are aware of the striking continuities between the viewpoints and diagnostic categories of colonial psychiatry and of contemporary health practitioners working in the Italian public system with migrants. The debates that most animate ethnopsychiatry today remain inextricable from colonial and post-colonial situations where relationships of power between colonizers and colonized have produced certain interpretations of mental illness and cultural difference.

During colonial and decolonization times, psychiatry and psychology contributed to the processes of culturalizing racial representations and essentializing cultural difference. These processes still constitute a risk for ethno-psychiatric practice today. Several studies of indigenous populations conducted by psychologists and psychiatrists from the 1940s to the 1960s marked the birth of ethnopsychiatry and gave it a specific ideological tone. In the early 1950s, John Carothers' analysis of the Mau Mau anti-colonial movement in Kenya as a violent behavior whose matrices were cultural was one example of psychiatry's collaboration with the colonial power structure in order to understand indigenous mentalities and behaviors to better govern them (Carothers 1953). John Colin Carothers (1954) interpreted the Mau Mau's deviance and opposition to colonial governance as "traditional," as an expression of local "customs," or, in other instances, as a psychological reaction to the conflicts produced by the encounter with European powers and their ways of being "modern." In this way, the political dimension of these acts of resistance, and the historical subjectivity of the people involved in such movements, were completely leveled to the order of cultural difference or psychopathology. The construction of a racial and cultural stereotype of the African served to legitimize colonial power, as well as to reduce local movements of resistance to psychopathology (Collignon 1997; McCulloch 1995; Vaughn 2001). In the colonial context, psychiatry doubled its function of control by reducing historical dynamics, political revolts, and conscious acts of resistance to the existing colonial power to "symptoms" of various nature: a complex mix of dependency on the colonizer, conflicts deriving from the exposure to the colonizer's culture, and the speed of the transformation of traditional models into European ways of being "modern."

Other studies of the mental health of the colonized populations had very different political implications. Octave Mannoni in Madagascar and Frantz Fanon in Algeria, for example, were actively engaged in a radical critique of colonial power and the relationships of domination and racism established by it. Although sympathetic with the Malagasy rebellion against the colonizers, Mannoni interpreted the suffering and rage that followed the imposition of forced labor and the Malagasy revolt in psychopathological terms as "the congruence of two personality crises" (Bloch in Mannoni 1990: xi). He identified the dialectic between the "inferiority complex" of the colonizer and the "dependency complex" of the colonized as the underlying dynamic that defined their relationship. According to this dialectical relation, Europeans projected their fears onto the local populations while the Malagasy, in turn, projected onto the whites a dependency that mirrored their relationship to their ancestors and the hierarchical religious structure according to which the dead represented a moral authority (Cole 2001; Roudinesco 2005). While the Malagasy saw in the "colonial fathers" the equivalent of their ancestors who protected and dominated them, the colonizers interpreted this form of dependency as an expression of the black's inferiority and subordination to their rule. According to Mannoni, the colonizer translated the Malagasy sense of dependency into an inferiority complex in order to legitimize the relationship of domination and abuse of the colonial power.

Ethnographies of colonialism have shown how colonial encounters were characterized by a tragic comedy of errors and misunderstandings in which each group's uncertainty about the other confirmed pre-existing anxiety and stereotypes (Mbembe 1997; Peel 2003; Obeyesekere 2005; Beneduce 2008). The nature of the misunderstanding at the root of Mannoni's interpretation brings us back to a crucial question in ethnopsychiatry: how is culture used and manipulated to make sense of difference, even in situations in which this very appeal to culture conceals rather than explains the dynamics of power and domination at the heart of conflicts? Maurice Bloch, writing on Mannoni's work, argued that the reason for this misunderstanding was Mannoni's arrogance:

> It is not the racist arrogance of the white man . . . . It is the arrogance of the psychoanalyst or anthropologist, who unthinkingly comes to indulge in the

> different but no less objectionable claim to superiority that his professional knowledge apparently gives him. . . . Ultimately, Mannoni disguises his ignorance of Malagasy motives only by substituting other motives deduced from theories originating in the highly specific intellectual tradition of his own culture. (Mannoni 1990: xviii–xix)

This is precisely the critique that, a few years after the publication of *Prospero and Caliban*, Frantz Fanon developed in *Black Skin, White Masks* ([1952] 1967) in order to respond to Mannoni's interpretation of the colonial encounter. Fanon argued that Mannoni reduced the conflicts between the colonizer and the colonized to a sophisticated psychological dynamic that kept the colonized in a position of dependency. While Fanon recognized the honesty of Mannoni's study of "the extreme ambivalence inherent in the colonial situation," he also denounced the tendency, characteristic of psychological research in general to lose sight of the real (Fanon [1952] 1967: 83).

Fanon contested the assumption that the origin of certain complexes was latent in the colonized from childhood and that the encounter with the colonizer only allowed it to manifest itself. This attempt to make the inferiority complex something that antedated colonization echoed psychiatry's mechanism of explanation according to which "[t]here are latent forms of psychosis that become overt as the result of a traumatic experience" (1967: 85). Instead, Fanon looked at the colonial situation both as the emergence of a particular encounter between "the white" and "the negro" that "only a psychological analysis [could] place and define" (85), and, most importantly, as the expression of racism that needed to be confronted from a militant position of denunciation rather than from a purely intellectual analytical position. Fanon wrote from the position of an engaged anti-colonialism, which he expressed in his writings and practice as a psychiatrist. He argued that the colonial encounter needed to be analyzed not only from its pathological roots, but also for its political, economic, and cultural implications.

Overall, colonial psychology and psychiatry tended to erase the political meaning of behaviors, struggles, movements of resistance, and rituals. Cultural difference was invoked in place of the political. In this context, the meanings of culture, along with its contradictions, paradoxes, and dynamics are often distorted. This same problem applies to the contemporary use of culture as a way to flatten the political dimension of suffering. Nevertheless, the colonial context also gave rise to the work of militant doctors like Frantz Fanon, who showed the interconnections of the political and cultural implications of suffering and domination. The Centro Fanon's clinical work is inscribed in this line of therapeutic and political intervention.

Culture: Therapeutic Trigger or Impossible Home?

In *Black Skin, White Masks,* Fanon denounces the trauma induced by the gaze of the colonizer on the colonized. Colonization creates a form of alienation experienced by the black man as an interior disintegration. The gaze of the white turns the body of the black into a speechless body, powerless in its silence: "I am being dissected under white eyes, the only real eyes. I am *fixed*" (Fanon [1952] 1967: 116). Overnight, Fanon writes, the Negro's customs and the sources on which they are based were wiped out "because they were in conflict with a civilization that he did not know and that imposed itself on him" (110). In *Toward the African Revolution* ([1964] 1967), Fanon explains that the consequences of this dialectic are the sense of guilt and inferiority experienced by the black man. In order to avoid feeling guilty and inferior, the oppressed gets caught in two possible patterns: he either proclaims his unconditional adoption of the new cultural models, or he irreversibly condemns his own culture.

Colonization produced a fracture in identity, something Fanon conceived as irreversible. This fracture echoes de Martino's "cultural apocalypses" and the experience of the "crisis of presence." Colonization, as a disruptive event, brought about the liquidation of the natives' systems of reference, cultural patterns, and ties to the past. This process causes alienation in the colonized who is reduced to the "inferior race" that denies itself by absorbing the convictions, doctrines, and attitudes of the "superior race" (Fanon [1964] 1967: 38). In the colonizer's language, this alienation appears under the name of assimilation. In the dialectic of non-recognition inscribed in the colonial encounter, the black self is a construction of the white man, and he is fixed in the image of himself that the white mirrors back to him. This process of mystification intrinsic to the colonial situation, produces simulacra of the past, of the disappeared culture of the colonized, which becomes inaccessible precisely because it is reduced to a lifeless copy of itself.

What does it mean, for Fanon, to get disentangled from the web of alienation produced by the colonizer's gaze? Emancipation from the perverse relationship established by colonialism cannot happen through a return to origins. There is no culture, custom, or tradition to go back to because they have been obliterated by the white man. To become emancipated by the colonial situation one has to take responsibility for this fracture and start anew, free from the web of images and copies of one's self projected by the other, to create something different. "I am not a prisoner of history. I should not seek there for the meaning of my destiny. I should constantly remind myself that the real *leap* consists in introducing invention into existence" (Fanon [1954] 1967: 229).

Fanon interprets all ties to the past or attempts to recuperate a relationship to the origins as still other moments of alienation that repeat the process of becoming stranger to one's self. Freedom is attained by rejecting the system of domination, and it implies another rupture, almost a second act of self-effacement and self-destruction. The search for emancipation in the past is a "retroactive operation" that encases man in "the culture put into capsules" (Fanon [1964] 1967: 42). This process is not a creative act of re-appropriating one's own origins, but a further act of self-destruction because that culture has been destroyed and erased by the domination of the white man. In order for the revolution to happen, African people must not be guided by the past, but by the present and the future.[13]

When I asked Roberto Beneduce why he named the ethnopsychiatric center after Fanon, he explained that the similarities between the increased numbers of documented and undocumented migrants in Italy in the early 1990s and the colonial situation described by Fanon was so striking that his name imposed itself on a clinic whose goal was to bring together political engagement and clinical intervention for post-colonial populations facing different forms of institutional racism. "The figure of Fanon seemed central to me, not as a metaphor or as a rhetorical image, but because he had succeeded in bringing together the contributions of psychoanalysts with the historic problems of language."[14]

Fanon's work had a great appeal to the group of ethno-psychiatrists and cultural mediators led by Beneduce in the late 1990s for several reasons. First, Fanon's reflection on the colonial situation allowed them to frame the issues related to migrants' mental health within the frame of the post-colonial and psychiatry's colonial legacy. Moreover, Fanon provided a method to think about the relationships between psychoanalysis, history and subjectivity, and to address simultaneously the socio-historic and psychic dimensions of experience as contingencies that have an impact on people's being in the world.

Along with Fanon's work, Tobie Nathan's clinical work with migrants in the outskirts of Paris and his writings on therapy are also central to the Centro's clinical work. At the Centre George Devereux, Nathan and his team designed a form of therapy for migrants and their families that included their own systems of classification of mental illness. Nathan was influenced by Devereux's approach to the relationship between culture and psychiatry according to which "bare facts" always belong to at least two different discourses that complement each other but can never be held simultaneously (Devereux 1978). Ethnopsychiatry positions itself at the intersections of psyche and culture and explores the frontiers between the two without trying to explain one level of discourse in terms of the other. Ellen Corin has pointed out that for Devereux and Nathan, "culture and psyche are doublets or homological structures containing the same basic elements governed by analogous mechanisms" (Corin 1997: 347).

Clinical work with migrants raises the problem of what therapeutic techniques and theories are appropriate to apply. Since patients and therapists do not typically share the same therapeutic and epistemological frame, it becomes crucial to find a "space of mediation" in which to negotiate a common therapeutic frame. Nathan introduced the idea of organizing therapeutic groups composed of multiple professionals: Western mental health practitioners trained in psychoanalysis, practitioners from other parts of the world who speak the patients' language and are familiar with healing practices of their countries of origins, and cultural mediators (Nathan 2003: 68). The composition of the therapeutic group is aimed at facilitating the move from one etiological theory to another without interrupting the flow of speech within the therapeutic setting. The idea underlying this therapeutic strategy is that how patients position themselves vis-à-vis cultural material, how they manipulate and re-interpret it, has diagnostic and prognostic implications. Moreover, acknowledging the legitimacy and epistemological accuracy of other cultural interpretations (other than the ones articulated in Western conceptions of mental health) has proved to ease the patient's speech and unlock associative chains that contextualize symptoms within a personal and collective history (Corin 1997). This approach prevents the patient from getting caught in one hegemonic discourse on suffering provided by Western psychiatry.

In this therapeutic setting, Western mental health practitioners, practitioners from the patient's country of origin, and cultural mediators collaborate in the definition of the diagnosis. The presence of a mental health practitioner from the patient's country aims at recreating a familiar cultural environment to facilitate the expression of the symptoms, and allows use of the patient's mother tongue. Other ways of knowing and treating mental disorders among migrants are incorporated into the ethnopsychiatry session. Magico-religious practices such as prayers, healing through protective amulets, exorcism, and chanting of devotional songs are an integral part of the treatment.

One of the central themes in Nathan's work is the metaphor of culture as the womb. The womb contains and protects, but it eventually expels and forces us into a relationship with alterity, with the world other than the mother. In this sense, the womb is a space that articulates ambivalences having to do with confronting alterity, the other from the mother. For Corin, the metaphor of the womb allows us to think that "just as the psyche is protected by a 'membrane' regulating exchanges with the environment, identity is enveloped by a second structuring membrane framed by culture from the outside" (1997: 350). Displacement and migration can create a rupture in this "membrane" that facilitates the assignment of meaning to different experiences. In Nathan's work, the purpose of therapy is to reconstitute this structure by re-anchoring the patient within his cultural background.

In his later work, Nathan has continued to think about the containing and structuring functions of culture and how it can be applied as a therapeutic lever, but he departs from the metaphor of the womb and turns to that of traumatism as the frame through which symptoms are interpreted and treated. His approach to clinical work is generally more oriented toward the effectiveness of certain healing praxis than toward interpretation. The performance of rituals, the fabrication of objects and amulets, the recitation of sacred texts are more central than the interpretative process of unveiling meaning starting from the patient's words, silences, dreams, and *actes manqués*. The attempt to re-anchor the patient in their own cultural universe serves the purpose of re-inscribing symptoms within a frame that assigns them meaning and of reorienting the patient within what ethnopsychiatry figures as "tradition." "Symptoms are like text without context," Corin wrote, and therapy attempts to reconstruct the context within which symptoms appear coherent (1997: 352). In Nathan's work, this context is often referred to as the patient's "culture." Culture thus becomes a therapeutic tool for therapists. Reinserting the person into a cultural frame through eliciting traditional etiologies is thus the goal of therapy.

Nathan's conception of "culture" as a frame that can give coherence to experience differs considerably from Fanon's view that any attempt to return to an original culture is destined to reproduce alienation. I asked the ethnopsychiatrists at the Centro Fanon how much Nathan's model influenced their clinical practice and how they reconciled the divergent approaches to "culture" of Nathan and Fanon in the therapeutic encounter with migrant patients. In Beneduce's words:

> Nathan's model influenced the birth of the Centro Fanon and my approach towards my patients a great deal because the meaning of therapeutic trigger

> by way of cultural materials seemed extremely rich to me. When I say "therapeutic trigger of cultural material"—an expression from Devereux—I am referring to the waterfall of psychic and relational events that I saw emerging in the moment in which, with my patients I could evoke situations, say in Africa, which I had been able to personally explore in my work there. And they were events that multiplied every time I would evoke metaphors, places that they knew, that they had heard of, political figures from their national histories, references to people that were familiar to them. There was a kind of radical shift in the therapeutic scene.

While Nathan's psychoanalytic background strongly informs his approach to the ethnopsychiatric setting, he also believes that psychoanalysis is a hegemonic discourse not always apt to understand the complexities of patients' cultural backgrounds. In the book *Médecins et sorciers* (Nathan and Stengers 1996), Nathan contrasts psychoanalysis with traditional healers' thinking, which he considers to be more open to difference and able to re-orient the patient within a signifying frame.

Overall, Nathan is interested in the effectiveness of what takes place in therapy, in the processes of influence and suggestion, which get activated within the therapeutic setting. In *L'influence qui guérit*, he argues that "the psychoanalytic apparatus, by its very organization, triggers processes governed by analogy," even when the participants are not aware of it (Nathan 1994: 120). The material setting itself—the objects used, the words pronounced, the rituals performed, the languages used—can produce more transformations in the patient than psychoanalytic theories of the unconscious and transference. The power of perfomativity inherent in rituals and words is at the core of the healing process. For Nathan, healing takes place when the therapist is able to inhabit different systems of thought and draw from different traditions of healing, and the patient is re-inscribed within his own belief system.

The paradox of Nathan's project lies in several aspects of his work. While on the one hand he describes the ethnopsychiatric setting as a "space of mediation" that allows migrant patients to negotiate their multiple belongings to different cultures and to re-articulate their relationship vis-à-vis "home," on the other hand, he also engages in a project of re-anchoring patients within their past cultural traditions, regardless of the experiences of migration and rupture with that specific past. Therefore, the ethnopsychiatric setting seems to mirror the polysemic and fragmentary nature of migrants' experiences and reference points; in this sense Nathan assumes a dynamic concept of culture as a domain in constant transformation. Nonetheless, the therapeutic strategy of referring patients back to their "culture" implies a static idea of culture as a homogeneous placeholder of meanings, behaviors, beliefs, and conceptions of health and illness. This second aspect of Nathan's conceptualization of culture is at odds with current anthropological debates and critique of the concept of culture. Anthropology's conception of the dynamic dimension of culture according to which conservation and creativity, continuity and rupture coexist tends to be overshadowed by Nathan's clinical application of this concept. A more dynamic approach to culture allows for new notions of the individual to emerge, one who is both embedded in tradition while at the same time rupturing and transforming it. The experience of displacement often intensifies the tensions between continuity and transformation, and exposes individuals to an often-challenging negotiation between what is perceived as "tradition" and what is encountered as "new."

One of the ethnopsychiatrists at the Fanon Center explained to me that in her clinical work the concept of "culture" was something extremely complex to utilize and that the difficulty lay in the impossibility of analyzing the clinical encounter according to a perspective that was simultaneously anthropological and clinical. She believed that when therapists used culture as a clinical tool, they got caught in a series of complex processes of reification, manipulation, and re-articulation of the concept. She explained to me that in some consultations it is necessary to essentialize the idea of culture in order to bring the patient back to certain stereotypes and homogenizing ideas of culture in order to create—or re-create—a structure within which one can find points of reference. Nonetheless, she added that in other cases, it is crucial to deconstruct the very idea of culture and free patients from culturally shaped forms of identification. Since ethnopsychiatrists at the Centro Fanon are also trained as anthropologists, they are faced with the dilemma of how to reconcile or keep separate the anthropological critique of culture and its clinical application. Do these orders of reflection belong to radically different ontologies, or can they inform each other? In the ethnopsychiatrist's words, such friction cannot find an ultimate resolution and functions as a reminder for practitioners of the necessity of going back and forth, from the anthropological to the clinical and vice versa. In the clinic there can be moments when essentializing takes place, and it may be soon after followed by a moment of deconstruction. These are different phases of ethnopsychiatric work all aimed at helping the patient create his/her own position within cultural representations and identifications.

The risk of Nathan's model is that, by focusing on cultural otherness and on the importance of traditional etiologies, the socio-economic causes and consequences of migration are neglected. While his approach includes a critique of the public health system, which refuses the foreigner access, and an attack on psychiatric knowledge unable to account for cultural difference, it inevitably risks naturalizing and reifying cultural otherness. Didier Fassin (2000) has strongly criticized French ethnopsychiatry as a legacy of colonial psychiatry that still fosters the creation of ghettos in line with the republican idea of citizenship. He sees the practice of Nathan's ethnopsychiatry as a way to create a model of government that mirrors the colonial endeavor to control and marginalize the colonized in the name of scientific knowledge and clinical intervention (Fassin 2000: 238). I believe that ethnopsychiatry as practiced at the Centro Fanon opens up spaces of therapeutic intervention that are more complex than what Fassin portrays in the French context. It is not about creating ghettos, even though this may be one possible drift of ethnopsychiatry. In my ethnography, practitioners seemed to explicitly distance themselves from the lack of awareness of the political and social dimensions of migration that constitutes Fassin's main critique of Nathan's work. Beneduce once explained to me that in his clinical work it was crucial to foreground the suffering of the migrant as a political experience embedded in colonial and post-colonial experiences:

> It is the patients, in a way, who ask me not to forget the fact that they don't have a passport, a job, or that they feel looked upon with disdain by the authorities, or by the social workers, or by the population, that they weren't able to feel comfortable when they were in France or in England because they remembered what their grandparents had told them about the colonial experience. That history and their current precarious position represent variables which are just as important as the cultural ones on which Nathan had constructed his fascinating work.

Working from within the tensions and contradictions of Fanon's reflections on culture and Nathan's use of the same concept creates a space for thinking critically about relationships of domination and their consequences for mental health and healing. The combination of these approaches minimizes the tendency to reify culture on the one hand and, on the other, to reduce culture to a ruin of the past that is unattainable in the present. At the Centro Fanon, practitioners are inspired by Nathan's model of therapy inasmuch as the effectiveness of symbols and etiologies from the patient's cultural background are taken seriously, and culture is considered therapeutic inasmuch as it provides a context wherein symptoms acquire meaning for the migrant.

While for Nathan the political dimension of suffering is in the background of his clinical work and he mainly focuses on the deconstruction of diagnostic criteria without looking at the larger implications of migration in the lives of the patients, Fanon's lesson forces us to face the concrete ways migrants are marginalized and suspended in a constant threat of not being recognized and legitimized within the receiving country. Fanon's approach to clinical practice allows the group at the Centro to always position their practice within the field of the political, in the sense of a political critique not only of psychiatry as hegemonic discourse, but also of other ideological fields that influence the conditions of precariousness of migrants. The fact of not having a passport, a residency permit, or a job, constitutes an important variable in the clinical work, just as Nathan's analysis of cultural variables proves to be effective in curing patients. The challenge the Centro Fanon's group faces is to keep these two approaches together, in tension with each other, in the attempt to be vigilant concerning the risks inherent in either perspective and in the political context in which the encounter with the other takes place. As Beneduce has pointed out, this approach can be portrayed as "politico-therapy" (Beneduce 2007: 89).

Conclusion

Ethnopsychiatry is haunted by the practice of working with the "truth" of the other's "culture." This effort is often fraught with an ambivalence that concerns, on the one hand, the desire to recuperate the lost memory of the other. This urge to redeem the migrant's alterity—which is often made invisible in dominant discourses on mental health—is fundamental in ethnopsychiatry's counter political project aimed at restoring the often-misrecognized archive of the colonized, and the marginal. On the other hand, this project's ambivalence reveals itself when the very recognition of the other's difference evokes discomfort and anxiety in patients themselves. When "culture" is invoked outside of the original context for the purpose of including migrants within the boundaries of the receiving country, a complex process of inscription and assignment of difference occurs. It has not been the purpose of this chapter to outline what elsewhere I define as the "persecutory dimension of culture" (Giordano 2008), but I have tried to clarify the risk in ethnopsychiatric practice of reifying the idea of "culture" without much reflection on the resistances that patients may have for representations of "home." What figures as "culture" in the clinical encounter may refer to homes that have become inhospitable and haunted by memories of violence and rupture and cannot be re-inhabited again, neither literally nor symbolically.

While the ethnopsychiatric project does constitute a political effort to question universalistic conceptions of mental health and healing by opening up a new field of practice in which cultural difference becomes central, there is the danger of objectifying culture as the exclusive domain of the other and as a fixed container of meanings that does not allow for a radical questioning of institutional discourses on mental health and difference. Rosalba Terranova-Cecchini, a leading figure in Italian transcultural psychiatry, has argued that current reflections on difference mainly serve the political debate about foreigners, foreclosing the opportunity to challenge the dominant scientific models and practices of Western psychiatry which, in fact, are influenced by transcultural processes (technological, scientific, ideological) (Terranova-Cecchini, 2002).

Terranova-Cecchini's critique points to what may be seen as a limit in ethnopsychiatry: the fact that it may not allow us to face the silence and hidden "truths" about ourselves, our own colonial archive and the various histories of Italian migration. By addressing the nexus of foreign migration and mental health exclusively, ethnopsychiatry risks avoiding questions about the estrangement from ourselves, and about difference within Italian society. What would it mean to regain access to one's own memory through the encounter with the migrant? How to access a repressed truth that comes back in a different form through the encounter with difference, to access the archive of Italian historical memory and identity, is another challenge that ethnopsychiatry needs to confront in order to fully exercise its political potential to interrupt dominant biomedical discourses and create difference from within.

Cristiana Giordano is Associate Professor of Anthropology at the University of California, Davis. She received her Ph.D. from the University of California, Berkeley. Her book, *Migrants in Translation: Caring and the Logics of Difference in Contemporary Italy* (University of California Press, 2014), won the Victor Turner Book Prize for ethnographic writing (2016) and the Boyer Prize in Psychoanalytic Anthropology (2017). Her current research investigates new ways of rendering ethnographic material into artistic forms. She has been collaborating with playwright and director Greg Pierotti on a new methodology at the intersection of the social sciences and performance. They have created *Unstories*, a 50-minute performance around the current "refugee crisis" in Europe, and *Unstories II (roaming)*, a 45-minute performance that furthers the reflection about movement and borders.

Notes

1. At the time of my research between 2002 and 2004, the Centro Fanon received funding from the municipality, the Province, Ministry of Health, and the European Community.
2. These questions animate contemporary Italian debates on difference and mental health as they are developed in a series of journals. Among these, the I Fogli di ORISS emerged as part of the work of the Organizzazione Interdisciplinare Sviluppo e Salute (Interdisciplinary organization for development and health, www.oriss.org), a non-profit that was founded in 1990 by a group of researchers and practitioners interested in the intersections of anthropology, medicine, psychiatry, and psychology, and engaged in development projects on health and therapies in Italy and abroad. *Antropologia Medica,* the Italian Medical Anthropology Society (SIAM) journal founded in the late 1980s, is another site where these debates have been developed (http://www.antropologiamedica.it/am.html). In 1988, *La Ricerca Folklorica,* devoted one issue to ethnopsychiatry (http://www.grafo.it/html/scheda_folklore.asp?IDFolklore=17). In the 1980s, the issues of foreign migration to Italy and the challenges it posed to Italian institutions were beginning to come to the foreground of political and medical debates, and, within academia, of theoretical conversations about the relationship to alterity and its consequences on integration policies. In the 1990s, new services and therapeutic models started to be implemented inside and outside state institutions. The Centro Fanon emerged in this political and theoretical climate, along with other similar attempts to respond to the new demands.
3. Roberto Beneduce is one of the leading figures in Italian ethnopsychiatry and also the founder of the Frantz Fanon Center. He practiced for many years as a psychiatrist in the public health care system, and founded the Center in 1996. He also trained in medical anthropology and joined the department of anthropology at the University of Turin (Italy). He conducts field research in Mali and Cameroon and practices as an ethnopsychiatrist at the Fanon Center. In Italy, other clinicians and medical anthropologists who have been engaged in debates about ethnopsychiatry and transcultural psychiatry are: Simona Taliani (2006), Francesco Vacchiano (2006), Mariella Pandolfi (1990; 2005), Rosalba Terranova-Cecchini (1990), Tullio Seppilli (1989), Goffredo Bartocci (1998), Luigi Frighi (1992), Alfredo Ancora (1997), Pino Schirripa (1990; 2005), Giuseppe Cardamone (1990; 1996), Salvatore Inglese (1989; 1997), Piero Coppo (1996; 2005), Pompeo Martelli (2005; 2006; 2009), and Natale Losi (2000).
4. Although concrete responses in the form of culturally specific services for migrant patients started to emerge in the early and mid-1990s, the terrain for this therapeutic work had emerged earlier as a theoretical problem. In 1984, within the School of Psychiatry at the University of Rome, Mariella Pandolfi and others founded the first Society of Transcultural Psychiatry as part of the Italian Psychiatric Society. Around the same time, in the context of the international conference of the Psychiatric Association, Pandolfi organized a workshop on transcultural therapies that gathered important scholars and practitioners from different parts of the world. Among others, Ellen Corin, Gilles Bibeau, and Tobie Nathan were introduced to the Italian context. Pandolfi was instrumental in bringing different schools of thought around transcultural mental health to Italy, specifically the North American schools of Harvard and Montreal, and the French school of Nathan (Giordano 2005).
5. In 1979, Tobie Nathan, psychologist and psychoanalyst of Jewish Egyptian origins, participated in the establishment of the first ethnopsychiatric clinic with Georges Devereux. In 1988, he founded the Centre Georges Devereux, an ethnopsychiatric center for mi-

grants linked to the Université Paris VII in Saint-Denis, in the periphery of Paris. He named the center after his teacher Georges Devereux from whom he had taken distance, both theoretically and clinically.

6. From the documentary by Sergio Zavoli entitled *I giardini di Abele*, produced in 1968 for the TV7 channel (quoted in Giannichedda 2005: XXXI).
7. The closest translation of *manicomio* into English is "mental hospital" or "asylum."
8. Interview conducted and recorded by the author in Turin, Italy, on 6 October 2003.
9 From the same interview conducted and recorded by the author in Turin, Italy, on 6 October 2003.
10. At the time of my fieldwork in Italy (2002–2004), the reform draft sponsored by the center-right Forza Italia deputy Maria Burani Procaccini during the right-wing government in 2001–2005 essentially promoted a discourse that described mentally ill patients as subjects dangerous to themselves and to society in need of control and discipline. From this viewpoint, a "cure" becomes compulsory and therapy is replaced with control. For a more updated account of mental health services in Italy and Basaglia's legacy, see Martelli and Cottino (2006).
11. This and the following quotes from Beneduce are translated from interviews conducted and recorded by the author in Turin, Italy, on 21 March and 3 July 2003.
12. The anti-psychiatry movement, and Basaglia in particular, had a complex relationship with the Italian Communist Party. Giovanni Berlinguer, a major figure in the party at that time, visited the hospital in Gorizia and remained an important mediator between Basaglia's ideas and the Communist Party (Giannichedda 2005: xxiii). Although Basaglia's political alliances within the party played an important role in the reform of the mental health system, he also interpreted the relationship between reality, ideology, and utopia in a way that differed from a certain revolutionary culture of leftist movements and from the party's program of reform. For these reasons, Basaglia is sometimes described as the solitary leader of the anti-institutionalization and anti-psychiatry movement that recognized him as a leader but that only partially shared his vision (Giannichedda 2005: xxx).
13. In *Towards the African Revolution*, Fanon takes a more complex position vis-à-vis the role of the past in providing tools for the revolution. He writes: "Rediscovering tradition, living it as a defense mechanism, as a symbol of purity, of salvation, the decultured individual leaves the impression that the mediation takes vengeance by substantializing itself. This falling back on archaic positions having no relation to technical development is paradoxical. The institutions thus valorized no longer correspond to the elaborate methods of action already mastered. . . . This rediscovery, this absolute valorization almost in defiance of reality, objectively indefensible, assumes an incomparable and subjective importance. On emerging from these passionate espousals, the native will have decided . . . to fight all forms of exploitation and of alienation of man. At this same time, the occupant, on the other hand, multiplies appeals to assimilation, then to integration, to community. . . . The plunge into the chasm of the past is the condition and the source of freedom. The logical end of this will to struggle is the total liberation of the national territory. In order to achieve this liberation, the inferiorized man brings all his resources into play, all his acquisitions, the old and the new, his own and those of the occupant" ([1964] 1967: 42–43).
14. Interview conducted and recorded by the author in Turin, Italy, on 21 March 2003.

References

Ancora, Alfredo. 1997. *La Dimensione Transculturale della Psicopatologia: Uno Sguardo da Vicino* [Transcultural Dimension of Psychopathology: A Close-up]. Rome: Edizioni Universitarie Romane.

Bartocci, Goffredo, and Raymond Prince. 1998. "Pioneers in Transcultural Psychiatry: Ernesto de Martino (1908–1965)." *Transcultural Psychiatry* 35(1): 111–23.

Basaglia, Franco. 1968. *L'Istituzione Negata* [The Denied Institution]. Turin: Einaudi.

———. 1981. *Scritti, 1953–1968* [Writings, 1953-1968]. Turin: Einaudi.

———. 2005. *L'utopia della Realtà* [The Utopia of Reality]. Turin: Einaudi.

Beneduce, Roberto. 1998. *Frontiere dell'Identità e delle Memoria. Etnopsichiatria e Migrazioni in un Mondo Creolo* [Frontiers of Identity. Ethnopsychiatry and Migrations in a Kreole World]. Milan: Franco Angeli.

———, ed. 2005. *Antropologia della Cura* [Anthropology of Care]. Turin: Bollati Boringhieri.

———. 2007. *Etnopsichiatria: Sofferenza Mentale e Alterità fra Storia, Dominio e Cultura* [Ethnopsychiatry: Mental Suffering and Alterity between History, Domination and Culture]. Rome: Carocci.

———. 2008. "L'Écoute de la Souffrance chez les Immigrés ou l'Histoire comme Symptôme" [Listening to Suffering among Migrants or History as Symptom]. *Confluences* 21: 22–25.

Beneduce, Roberto, and Pompeo Martelli. 2005. "Politics of Healing and Politics of Culture: Ethnopsychiatry, Identities and Migration." *Transcultural Psychiatry* 42(3): 367–93.

Callieri, Bruno. 2001. *Quando Vince l'Ombra: Problemi di Psicopatologia Clinica* [When Shadow Prevails: Issues in Clinical Psychopathology]. Rome: Edizioni Universitarie Romane.

Cardamone, Giuseppe, and Pino Pini. 1996. "Risorse comunitarie e salute mentale" [Community Based Resources and Mental Health]. *I Fogli di ORISS* 5: 57–78.

Cardamone, Giuseppe, and Pino Schirripa. 1990. "Lo Colio e la Salvezza: Un Culto Terapeutico in Calabria" [Colio and Salvation: A Therapeutic Cult in Calabria]. *Daedalus* 4: 127–45.

Carothers, John Colin. 1953. *The African Mind in Health and Disease: A Study in Ethnopsychiatry*. Geneva: World Health Organization.

———. 1954. *The Psychology of Mau Mau*. Nairobi: Printed by the Govt. Printer.

Cole, Jennifer. 2001. *Forget Colonialism? Sacrifice and the Art of Memory in Madagascar*. Berkeley: University of California Press.

Collignon, René. 1997. "Aliénation Mentale et Altérité du Sujet Colonial: De quelques Difficultés de l'Émergence d'une relation Thérapeutique Basée sur le Dialogue en Afrique" [Mental Alienation and the Alterity of the Colonial Subject: On the Challeges of a Therapeutic Relationship Based on Dialogue in Africa]. In *Saperi, linguaggi e tecniche nei sistemi di cura tradizionali* [Knowledges, anguages and echniques in traditional systems of cure]. ed. Roberto Beneduce, 71–88. Turin: L'Harmattan Italia.

Coppo, Piero. 1996. *Etnopsichiatria* [Ethnopsychiatry]. Milan: Il Saggiatore.

———. 2005. *Le Ragioni del Dolore: Etnopsichiatria della Depressione* [The Reasons of Pain: Ethnopsychiatry of Depression]. Turin: Bollati Boringhieri.

Corin, Ellen. 1997. "Playing with Limits: Tobie Nathan's Evolving Paradigm in Ehnopsychiatry." *Transcultural Psychiatry* 34(3): 345–58.

de Martino, Ernesto. 1941. *Naturalismo e Storicismo nell'Etnologia* [Naturalism and Historicism in Ethnology]. Bari: Laterza.

———. 1956. "Crisi della Presenza e Reintegrazione Religiosa" [The Crisis of Presence and Religious Reintegration]. *Aut Aut 31*: 17–38.

———. 1977. *La Fine del Mondo: Contributo all'Analisi delle Apocalipsi Culturali* [The End of The World: Contributions to the Analysis of Cultural Apocalypses]. Turin: Einaudi.
———. 2000 (1948). *Il Mondo Magico. Prolegomani a una Storia del Magismo* [Magic World. Prolegomena to a History of Magic]. Turin: Bollati Boringhieri.
Devereux, George. 1978. *Ethnopsychoanalysis: Psychoanalysis and Anthropology as Complementary Frames of Reference*. Berkeley: University of California Press.
Fanon, Frantz. (1952) 1967. *Black Skin, White Masks*. New York: Grove Press.
———. (1963). *The wretched of the earth: A negro psychoanalyst's study of problems of racism and colonialism in the world today*. New York, NY: Grove Press.
———. (1964) 1967. *Towards the African Revolution (Political Essays)*. New York: Grove Press.
Fassin, Didier. 2000. "Les Politiques de l'Ethnopsychiatrie: La Psyché Africaine, des Colonies Britanniques aux Banlieues Parisiennes" [Politics of Ethnopsychiatry: The African Psyche, from British Colonies to the Parisian Peripheries]. *L'Homme* 153: 231–50.
Foucault, Michel. 1961. *Histoire de la Follie à l'Âge Classique* [The Hisotry of Madness]. Paris: Plon.
———. 1994. "Psychiatric Power." In *Ethics, Subjectivity and Truth*, ed. Paul Rabinow, 39–50. New York: The New Press.
Frighi, Luigi. 1992. "Le Problematiche Trans-Culturali in Psichiatria e in Igiene Mentale" [Transcultural Issues in Psychiatry and Mental Health Services]. In *Cultura Malattia Migrazioni: La Salute degli Immigrati Extracomunitari in Italia ed in Campania: Aspetti Sociali, Medici e Psicologici* [Cultura Illness Migrations: Immigrants' Health in Italy and Campania], ed. Alfredo Dama, Tommaso Esposito, and Teresa Arcella. Regione Campania USL 27: Dipartimento di Salute Mentale, Pomigliano D'Arco.
Giannichedda, Maria Grazia. 2005. "L'Utopia della Realtà: Franco Basaglia e L'Impresa della sua Vita" [Utopia of Reality: Franco Basaglia and his Life's Mission]. In *L'Utopia della Realtà* [Utopia of Reality], by Franco Basaglia, VII–LII.Turin: Einaudi.
Giordano, Cristiana. 2005. "Intervista a Mariella Pandolfi" [Mariella Pandolfi: an Interview]. *Passaggi: Rivista Italiana di Scienze Transculturali* [Passages: Italian Review of Transcultural Sciences] 7.
———. 2008. "Practices of Translation and the Making of Migrant Subjectivities in Contemporary Italy." *American Ethnologist* 35(4): 588–606.
Goffman, Erving. 1961. *Asylums: Essays on the Social Situation of Mental Patients and Other Inmates*. New York: Anchor Books.
Inglese, Salvatore, and Barbara Madia. 1989. "Ideologia della Morte, Tecniche Rituali e Immaginario Collettivo a San Giovanni in Fiore" [Ideology of Death, Ritual Techniques and Collective Imaginary in San Giovannin in Fiore]. *Daedalus* 2: 108–50.
Inglese, Salvatore, and Cesare Peccarisi. 1997. *Psichiatria Oltre Frontiera: Viaggio intorno alle Sindromi Culturalmente Ordinate* [Psychiatry beyond the Border: Journey around Culturally Bound Syndroms]. Milan: UTET Periodici.
Jervis, Giovanni. 1994. *La Psicoanalisi Come Esercizio Critico* [Psychoanalysis as Critical Exercise]. Milan: Garzanti.
Keller, Richard C. 2007. *Colonial Madness: Psychiatry in French North Africa*. Chicago: University of Chicago Press.
Kirmayer, Laurence. 1999. "Myth and Ritual in Psychotherapy." *Transcultural Psychiatry*, 36(4): 451–60.
Losi, Natale. 2000. *Vite Altrove: Migrazione e Disagio Psichico* [Lives Elsewhere: Migrations and Psychic Distress]. Milan: Feltrinelli Editore.

Mannoni, Octave. 1990. *Prospero and Caliban: The Psychology of Colonization*. Ann Arbor: University of Michigan Press.
Martelli, Pompeo. 2009. "Working Together for Public Health." *Transcultural Psychiatry* 46(2): 316–27.
Martelli, Pompeo, and Gaia Cottino. 2006. "The Age of Anxiety: Stones, Feathers and Re-institutionalization." *Anthropology & Medicine* 13(3): 265–71
Mbembe, Achille. 1997. *La Naissance du Maquis dans le Sud-Cameroun (1920–1960)* [The Birth of the Maquis in Southern Cameroun (1920-1960)]. Paris: Karthala.
McCulloch, Jock. 1995. *Colonial Psychiatry and the "African Mind."* Cambridge: Cambridge University Press.
Nathan, Tobie. 1994. *L'Influence qui Guérit* [The Curing Influence]. Paris: Odile Jacob.
———. 2003. *Non Siamo Soli al Mondo* [We are not Alone in the World]. Turin: Bollati Boringhieri.
Nathan, Tobie, and Isabelle Stengers. 1996. *Médicins et Sorciers* [Doctors and Healers]. Paris: Odile Jacob.
Obeyesekere, Gananath. 2005. *Cannibal Talk: The Man-Eating Myth and Human Sacrifice in the South Seas*. Berkeley: University of California Press.
Pandolfi, Mariela. 1990. "Boundaries Inside the Body: Women's Suffering in Southern Peasant Italy." *Culture, Medicine and Psychiatry* 14(2): 255–74.
Pandolfi, Mariella, and Gilles Bibeau. 2005. "Souffrance, Politique, Nation: Une Cartographie de L'Anthropologie Médicale Italienne" [Suffering, Politics, Nation: A Map of Italian Medical Anthropology]. In *Anthropologie Médicale: Ancrages Locaux, Défits Globaux* [Medical Anthropology: Local Anchors, Global Challenges]. ed. Francine Sailant and Serge Genest, 199–232. Montreal, Quebec: Presse de l'Université Laval.
Peel, John David Yeadon. 2003. *Religious Encounters and the Making of the Yoruba*. Bloomington: Indiana University Press.
Rechtman, Richard. 2000. "Stories of Trauma and Idioms of Distress: From Cultural Narratives to Clinical Assessment." *Transcultural Psychiatry* 37(3): 403–15.
Risso, Michele, and Wolfgang Böker. 1992. *Sortilegio e Delirio: Psicopatologia dell'Emigrazione in Prospettiva Transculturale* [Spell and Delirium: Psychopathology of Emigration from a Transcultural Perspective]. Napoli: Liguori Editore.
Roudinesco, Elisabeth. 2005. "Decolonizzare se stessi" [Decolonize One's Self]. In *Etnopsicoanalisi: Temi e Protagonisti di un Dialogo* Incompiuto [Ethnopsychoanalysis: Themes and Protagonists of an Unfinished Dialogue]. ed. Roberto Beneduce, Bertrand Pulman, and Elisabeth Roudinesco, 129–38. Turin: Bolati Boringhieri.
Saunders, George R. 1993. "'Critical Ethnocentrism' and the Ethnology of Ernesto de Martino." *American Anthropologist* 95(4): 875–93.
Scheper-Hughes, Nancy, and Anne Lovell, eds. 1987. *Psychiatry Inside-Out: Selected Writings of Franco Basaglia*. New York: Columbia University Press.
Schirripa, Pino. 2005. *Politiche della Cura: Terapie, Potere e Tradizione nel Ghana Contemporaneo* [Politics of Care: Theapies, Power and Tradition in Contemporary Ghana]. Rome: Argo.
Seppilli, Tullio. 1989. *Medicine e Magie: Le Tradizioni Popolari in Italia* [Medicine and Magic: Popular Traditions in Italy]. Milan: Electa.
———. 2001. "Medical Anthropology 'At Home': A Conceptual Framework and the Italian Experience." *AM Rivista della Società italiana di antropologia medica* 11–12: 23–36.
Simons, Ronald C. 1996. *Boo! Culture, Experience, and the Startle Reflex*. Oxford, UK: Oxford University Press.

Taliani, Simona, and Francesco Vacchiano, eds. 2006. *Altri Corpi: Antropologia ed Etnopsicologia della Migrazione* [Other Bodies: Anthropology and Ethnopsychology of Migration]. Milan: Edizioni Unicopoli.

Terranova-Cecchini, Rosalba. 2002. "Intervista" [Interview]. *Passaggi: Rivista Italiana di Scienze Transculturali* [Passages: Italian Review of Transcultural Sciences] 2: 44–53.

Terranova-Cecchini, Rosalba, and Paolo Inghilleri. 1990. *Nuove frontiere della psicologia transculturale* [New frontiers of transcultural psychology]. Milan: Franco Angeli.

Vaughan, Megan. 1991. *Curing their Ills: Colonial Power and African Illness.* Cambridge: Polity Press.

Wazir, Jahan Karim, ed. 1990. *Emotions of Culture: A Malay Perspective.* Oxford, UK: Oxford University Press.

Winzeler, Robert L. 1995. *Latah in Southeast Asia.* Cambridge, UK: Cambridge University Press.

5

Precarity, Chronic Illness, and Borders of Care Confronting Immigrants in Paris, France

Carolyn Sargent, Laurent Zelek, and Anne Festa

> In 2009, I discovered a lump in my right breasts and under my arm. I went to Kita (Mali) and the doctor said it was a lump. I thought it was a ball of fat. My sister made me a reservation at [a hospital in a large city]. There I had a biopsy and the doctor said that it was a cancer. I did not want to believe it. He did a biopsy and he said that it was a cancer. I had two sessions of chemotherapy . . . and my sister said I had to go to France for treatment. I managed to get a ticket and went to stay with a cousin. She took me to [a certain hospital] in Paris. There they told me that it was a cancer, that chemotherapy was necessary, then radiation, and surgery. When my cousin learned what I had, she refused to let me stay with her . . . an Association lodged me in a room in Paris. My husband has remarried . . . He wants nothing to do with me. The Association is helping me apply for papers. They made me enroll in training and I do housework. I cannot with my arm [swollen from surgery]. But I do it because I have to have a paycheck. The Association will help me apply for family reunification and bring my children to France.[1]
>
> —Foune, immigrant age 43, resident in Paris since 2009, breast cancer patient in treatment

France achieved global attention in 2000 when the World Health Organization rated the French health care system first in its quality rankings (Fassin 2004: 203). The French national health care system is highly centralized, established on a foundation of both public and private institutions. State policy and public sentiment reflect the ideological stance that health care is a human right and that national health insurance should eliminate financial barriers to medical care. In France, there does not exist (in theory) a situation where an indispensable treatment can be refused to a patient because of insufficient health coverage (except in the case of patients who are undocumented, and even in such instances, lack of care is rare). Ideologically, access to health care presents no obstacle to the sick.

Yet high life expectancy rates and other impressive health indicators notwithstanding, the French health care system has been critiqued for unequal access to health care for vulnerable and marginalized populations such as immigrants (Larchanché 2012). In contrast to the WHO rankings, the European Union noted dramatic gaps in health status in France by social class, especially by occupation. For the immigrant population of interest in this chapter, legal status—which affects access to employment, lodging, and health care—is equally significant in shaping access to health services and in constructing borders to care. As Pierre Aïach (2010, 2013; see also Standing 2011) observed, social inequalities have consequences that, in synergy, are progressively amplified. Accordingly, certain populations, in particular those living in economic precarity such as undocumented immigrants, are especially subject to health risks (Fassin 2004: 203). Low household revenue, unemployment, inadequate lodging, immigration status, and geographic locale may all influence health status and create borders limiting access to efficient and effective health care services. In addition, in response to the ongoing global economic crisis, austerity measures introduced across Europe, including in France, have increased existing inequalities in health care access for the most vulnerable populations (Cognet 2014; Fourmy 2013; Sargent and Kotobi 2017; Simonet 2013). Austerity in the health sector refers to reduction of government spending on public hospitals, health insurance coverage, unemployment compensation, and housing support for low-income households. Immigrants are systematically represented in the population at risk from state and regional institutional budget cuts affecting access to health services and quality of care.

In this chapter, we identify how these inequalities play out in everyday experiences of immigrant patients living with serious chronic illnesses such as cancer in the greater Paris metropolitan region and navigating borders to access health care. We identify the significance of the geospatial region in the distribution of and access to health resources, which is highly skewed in favor of major urban areas (Banki 2014). Accordingly, we focus on the much mediatized "immigrant suburb" of Seine-Saint-Denis, an administrative department annexed to northern and northeastern Paris (Insée 2011). We also identify the structures and dynamics that serve as borders constraining patients and their families from gaining access to health care facilities even when—in the abstract—they have the "right" to health care (Stuckler and Basu 2013; Torsoli 2013).

In the presence of life circumstances, which exacerbate the dilemmas posed by sickness itself, and in the absence of hospital services that can meet the needs of patients and their families, we suggest that associations independent of the hospital, usually state-subsidized but sometimes humanitarian or non-governmental, play an important role in offering advice and assistance (Jaouen 2015). Such interventions by associations such as those in Seine-Saint-Denis, for example, enable patients to remain in treatment for cancer, diabetes, or other serious conditions, while also addressing challenges posed by economic marginality and vulnerability. We will illustrate the important roles played by associations by focusing on one, AcSanté, situated in Seine-Saint-Denis, which is an exemplary model of health care provision for vulnerable patients such as low-income immigrants. Such associations work to deconstruct borders designed to restrict access to health care institutions and sources of social support, as two case studies will indicate.

National Health Policy: Oncology

Health policy in France, as part of a national health strategy (SNS, *Stratégie Nationale de Santé*), has the objective of guaranteeing the continuity, the coordination, and the quality of care offered to patients, as well as a homogeneous regional distribution of the offerings for prevention and care services. To guarantee this equity in health, the legislature has integrated into the law the notion of a health path. In order for this notion to be grasped by everyone, the idea is to assemble around a "shared strategy," capable of coming to the aid of those most in need.

In the particular case of oncology, the Cancer Plan 2 (INCa 2014) aimed, among other things, to reduce the inequalities facing illness, to help patients better their lives "before and after cancer." It also aimed to reduce clearly identified individual and environmental risk factors such as tobacco, alcohol, and diet. On 4 February 2014, a new, third cancer plan was presented. This plan aspires primarily to cure but also to help the patient and their family as well as to prepare for the future, regardless of social class: "To cure and to prevent cancer: we give the same opportunities to everyone, everywhere in France."

The objective to reduce inequalities, in other words, to reduce borders exiling prospective patients from care, takes on a particularly intense meaning in a territory like Seine-Saint-Denis, which concentrates these problems in one of the most populated territories (approximately 1.6 million inhabitants). According to the Regional Health Agency of Île-de-France (Projet Régional de Santé—PRS—2013/2017), Seine-Saint-Denis is considered the most structurally vulnerable department in the Paris metropolitan area, with an average income 30 percent below the average for the region. Approximately 11 percent of the population benefit from supplemental universal health coverage for the lowest income sector of the population (*Couverture Maladie Universelle complémentaire*), which represents the greatest proportion of any department in the greater Paris administrative area.

As of 31 December 2012, 144,854 beneficiaries of the family allowance fund (*Caisse d'Allocations Familiales*) were classified as low income, that is, with an income lower than 1,001 euros per month per "consumption unit." The population living in low-income households was estimated at 367,570 people, or 24.8 percent of the population of Seine-Saint-Denis, compared with 13.5 percent nationally. The department of Seine-Saint-Denis is therefore considered a sensitive territory in terms of poverty and precarity (*Zone Urbaine Sensible*, Sensitive Urban Zone). The social inequalities there are manifest in health inequities: for example, mortality from cancer is 4.5 times higher for men and twice as high for women compared with the most privileged in the department. An exhaustive analysis of population diversity in France (Beauchemin, Hamel, and Simon 2018) estimated that 66 percent of residents in Seine-Saint-Denis are immigrants, or children of immigrants.[2] Recently the French parliament suggested that between 150,000 and 300,000 undocumented migrants reside in the Seine-Saint-Denis department, although this estimate remains controversial (Chazan 2018).

Breast cancer is the primary cause of death from cancer among women in Seine-Saint-Denis, higher than the national average according to ORS (Observatoire Régionale de Santé 2013: 7.4.2.) Because of French government restrictions regarding data collection on ethnicity, race, and religion, it is difficult (if not impossible) to specify the numbers of cases of breast cancer among immigrants in Seine-Saint-Denis, or the differential mortality among populations by ethnicity or nationality of origin living in the Paris region. However, the data published by the regional health agency (Agence Régionale de Santé) and the regional health commission (*Observatoire Régional de Santé*) demonstrated that the situation of the inhabitants of Seine-Saint-Denis continue to deteriorate, notably in terms of the income gap compared with inner Paris. Access to health care for immigrants, especially those who are undocumented, is problematic, and depends on migrant understandings of their rights to health care coverage, among other factors that we will discuss below. These represent a borderland between those with national health coverage and supplemental private coverage, and those who are undocumented and thus have no legal right to health coverage except in emergency circumstances.

Seine-Saint-Denis is home to several hospitals that target low-income and immigrant populations; these include Hôpital Delafontaine and Hôpital Avicenne. These institutions served as primary sampling sites for Sargent's research on immigrants navigating the public health sector in the context of serious illness such as breast cancer (2014–2018). Laurent Zelek's professorial status at Avicenne and Delafontaine facilitated participant observation and collection of case studies, two of which are presented in this chapter (Zelek, Bodere, Bourlier, and Festa 2015). Anne Festa, then director of the association Oncologie93, also provided case material to enrich this discussion.

The organization of out-of-hospital care for the most precarious patients in the form of a health association, AcSanté (formerly Oncologie 93), facilitated provision of treatment and social support services for cancer patients undergoing treatment in Seine-Saint-Denis. The association comprised a network created in 2003, whose goal was to organize the collaboration between the different private and public health establishments in Seine-Saint-Denis. Secondarily, it pragmatically developed the establishment of "health paths." The health path is a concept that aims, through the coordination of actors from the health, social, and medico-social domains in connection with the patients and local authorities, to guarantee the continuity, accessibility, quality, security, and efficiency of care for the population. The health path takes into account geographical, demographic and seasonal specificities in each area, in order to reduce borders and barriers, and contribute to territorial equity.

AcSanté, for example, takes care of patients suffering from cancer and/or other serious chronic illnesses. It also takes care of the patients' families. The role of the network does not stop at clinical care during acute illness phases. Support continues well after the end of clinical interventions, as recommended by the Cancer Plan 2. The network allows for better coordination of care, for the evaluation of needs and/or the implementation of supportive care at home, at the office, but also for guidance and information concerning the illness and social and psychological support. This support and these evaluations of need are available as often as necessary during the illness trajectory.

The actions put in place by this network correspond to the axis of "living during and after cancer," which appears in the Cancer Plan 2, as well as to the very prominent guidance concerning the access to care for all and notably to supportive care for all. We find here the axes of the Cancer Plan 2, which are, among others, to prevent social deterioration, while combatting the inequalities of access to care and while specifically taking into account the most vulnerable populations, among these, immigrants living with minimal social and economic support.

One of the particularities of this network is to highlight the entanglement between precarity and health and the difficulties that certain patients—and here we focus on undocumented and vulnerable immigrants—can encounter in order to arrive at a "positive health path, given the impact of social difficulties on their care path. This leads to individualizing the notion of a complex situation within health paths, corresponding to a patient's state of health, disability, or social situation necessitating the intervention of several categories of professionals. For the most complex situations, the association leadership created a tool to encourage interactions among professionals; the tool also allows them to combine their different skills and expertise for the patient's benefit.

This group, known as the Social Dialogue Meeting (Réunion de Concertation Sociale), meets to address social dimensions of sickness that had previously been neglected with regard to patients living in precarity (immigrants, for instance). This population risks a deteriorating spiral based on the intersection between the biological (cancer, diabetes, kidney disease) and the social (lack of housing, unemployment, very low household revenue).

Measuring Precarity

Numerous scholars have explored the social determinants of health, yet in the context of associations whose mission is to stabilize the health and social well-being of immigrant patients, authorities—including Chief of Oncology at Avicenne and president of the association AcSanté, Laurent Zelek—sought to refine a scale of values, a score measuring precarity (Jaouen 2015; Sass et al. 2006). The objective of such a scale was to justify intervention in patient care and social support for some, rather than others. Funding agencies were especially intent on access to a quantitative instrument to validate providing financial support to the association and to particular patients. What difference in vulnerability exists, one might ask, between a young, isolated woman with a child suffering from breast cancer and an older person, with the same pathology, living in an apartment with little accessibility?

In 2011, the Oncologie 93 network (today AcSanté 93) responded to a call for projects (*Appel à projet*, AAP) of the regional health agency in order to obtain funding for the trial use of the EPICES score (*Évaluation de la précarité et des inégalités dans les centres d'examen de santé;* Evaluation of precarity and of inequalities in health examination centers). This instrument is a tracking tool for cancer patients (and/or their families) in a situation of social fragility and is intended to structure an evaluation subsequent to the cancer diagnosis. The hypothesis of this work was that identification of precarity at the time of cancer diagnosis would prevent its exacerbation during the course of treatment and thereafter.

This score was developed in 2002, following a study of 197,389 patients of health examination centers. These patients responded to eleven questions that summarize 90 percent of the features that constitute precarity of an individual. The interrelations between health, lifestyle, access to care and the two definitions of precarity were studied with logistic regression analyses. These analyses made it possible to choose eleven questions from among forty-two questions at the beginning. The sum of these eleven questions generate the EPICES score. The score is continuous. It varies from zero (absence of precarity) to one hundred (maximum of precarity). Precarity normally concerns those whose EPICES score is greater than forty. The statistical analysis showed that the EPICES score was ultimately a better indicator of precarity and of inequalities of health than precarity as defined in official texts. For example, if one begins with the assumption that the definition of precarity is only based on income level, some people will be considered non-precarious, even if their answers to the EPICES questionnaire present numerous signs of precarity. The evaluation of the EPICES score therefore enables a redefinition of the threshold of precarity, eventually lowered to 30.17 (basic level of the fourth quintile of the study).

The EPICES score presents the advantages of being individual, quantitative, easy to deliver and present, and of taking into account the multidimensional aspects of precarity. It also allows for health examination centers to monitor the patient population longitudinally. It has become an effective indicator for the association network, most particularly for alerting the coordination team about people experiencing social difficulties when a serious illness is diagnosed. Thus, the premise is that anticipating the needs of these patients and families can avoid an exacerbation of their situation, based on experience thus far.

The network for any care indicated also attends to those with an EPICES score below thirty. These people are simply in a less critical social and economic situation than those with a score above thirty. Their care is therefore less time consuming and sometimes necessitates less urgency in support and less investment from the team, since these people are often more autonomous and/or have more social support. However, it is sometimes possible that the care of a patient with a score lower than thirty is very important, notably concerning psychological or nutritional issues. Indeed, these (essentially medical) items are not "questioned" by means of the score in its present form. That is why the EPICES score remains solely an indicator and not an exclusive criterion of inclusion. It can help the network's coordination team identify the most fragile and the most urgent situations, which will necessitate anticipating care and alerting other health actors who might be involved in this care. However, it presents certain limits, and will not at all replace (nor will it contradict) the personal judgment of one of the members of the network, based on other criteria (psychological, psychiatric, cultural, medical, legal, and so forth).

The criteria for determining a complex situation for all cancer patients living in Seine-Saint-Denis and their immediate family include: a medical evaluation performed by the referring oncologist and/or the primary care physician ("serious" cancer and/or associated comorbidity and/or a pre-existing physical handicap and/or pre-existing addictions); a social evaluation, EPICES score >30 (in Seine-Saint-Denis indicates a precarious situation); a psychological evaluation revealing degrees of suffering including psychiatric conditions, a clinical evaluation interview by the psychological coordinator; and an evaluation of French language comprehension (assistance of an interpreter necessary for consultations).

These criteria for inclusion apply to immigrant patients suffering from cancer and to their families, but can apply to any impoverished population in great insecurity who are lost in the health system and for whom support, modeled on that used to take care of cancer, could be offered. Undocumented immigrants, and even immigrants legally residing in France, merit special attention because they may well lack documentation to facilitate access to clinical treatment and may also live at the limits of social precarity. Instability in residence, effect of treatment on capacity to work, decline in household revenue, difficulties obtaining childcare, may all converge with declining physical well-being to generate an unyielding border of constraint to care. Whereas hospitals are limited in offering measures to redress these problems, particularly with budget cuts and transformations in hospital management protocols (see Sargent and Kotobi 2017), associations such as AcSanté have a more flexible mandate. Primary to this mandate is the identification of patients living in extreme precarity; subsequently, an important objective is to demonstrate with validity how the social and the biological shape and reflect one another.

Social workers or psychologists associated with AcSanté generally elicit data for the Score EPICES. During the first interview, a person perceived as being in a situation of vulnerability might refuse to complete the Score EPICES and similarly might reject offers of support. The association network will then always propose a follow-up in the future and often at the moment of "spikes" in side effects from the treatments. This is scheduled to convey empathy with the patient when the psychological, medical, and social impact of the treatments and of the illness are felt most intensely. For those who are less vulnerable the follow-up will take place after the first chemotherapy sessions, more to take stock of potential side effects and assess access to supportive care. Concurrently, regular reports take place with professionals intervening at home, with the points of contact from the hospital, from associations and other institutions, and with the patient. These follow-ups are tailor-made for each situation.

No more than six months after putting personalized care in place, a new "scoring" takes place, to observe if the patient's situation has changed compared with the result of the first score. The higher the score, the more precarious the patient's status. A score that does not move in the right direction alerts those responsible to undertake another general overview with all of the participants in the clinical team, while obviously including the person concerned and their family. For example, for the question: "Do you benefit from supplemental health insurance?" in addition to the patient's answer, the network will verify that the other entitlements are well noted and open: update of entitlements, obtaining universal health coverage (CMU), state medical assistance for the undocumented (*Aide Médicale d'État*, AME), and so forth.

An Exemplary Case: Madame R

While this operational framework was in place, we met R. in April 2014. At the time, she was thirty-one years old, the mother of three young children, and living with advanced breast cancer. She had waited a year to seek care for breast pain, thinking a ritual specialist from her society of origin in West Africa might help. Eventually, she was referred to Professor Zelek, Head of Oncology at Avicenne Hospital.

The nurses in oncology proposed to her, early in her care, that the association team contact her to determine what forms of assistance she might need at home. The clinical team thought she needed help with her children, aged three to eleven, during the course of treatment.

Between April and May 2014, the association psychologist and the social worker were in telephone contact with her and begin to gather the administrative data to obtain help at home. They learned that the father of the children was present but could not be a constant source of support because he works at night rather far away in the suburbs.

R. did not respond to invitations to contact the association nor did her spouse. In July, the association was alerted after a meeting between Professor Sargent, who was conducting anthropological research on the unit, and Professor Zelek. R. was not attending her appointments regularly and had housing problems. A member of the anthropology team explained to the hospital nurses that R. could not have appointments for chemotherapy at the time when she needed to collect her child at school. This resulted in more convenient scheduling for subsequent appointments. Sargent and a cultural mediator visited R. at her home and learned that her landlord was harassing her. In addition, Professor Zelek and Sargent learned that her French residence permit was about to expire. It also became clear that although she had lived in France for ten years, she did not have health coverage (AME) for which she was eligible, because she was unaware of her rights.

In the meantime, immediately alerted by Prof. Zelek, the association took measures with the prefecture and with the CPAM (*Caisse Primaire d'Assurance Maladie*) to make sure that her rights to access care would not be interrupted. On 10 July 2014, R. agreed to a meeting with the network's team at her home, a one-bedroom apartment. R. described herself as extremely tired and brought up her concerns about the proprietor, who threatened her, and the rent. Her husband was absent because he worked long hours in a print shop. The association contacted him, and he explained that he was paying cash for the rent to stabilize the relationship with the proprietor.

The association proposed requesting housing in the locality where R. was then living with the children and writing to appropriate authorities in the city. At the same time, all involved were aware that access to housing in Seine-Saint-Denis is a serious problem and would involve a lengthy process.

Beginning in September, the "pressure" from the proprietor became more menacing and he threatened to break down the doors and force them to move. In the meantime, on separate occasions, the anthropologists, the cultural mediator, and the association representative returned to the home several times. All observed red spots on R.'s forearms, which itched; the youngest child was also scratching. The association arranged an emergency appointment for her at Avicenne, where she was diagnosed with scabies.

Between July and November 2014, R. was in regular contact with the association, every eight days on average, and with two anthropologists and an interpreter. Her Score EPICES, calculated by AcSanté, originally 81.66, was 70 after a six-month interval, a slight improvement but still problematic (score over forty indicates socioeconomic precarity). She received "support" for the legal-administrative situation: letters, renewed requests, checking with public authorities, with particular attention paid to the question of medical insurance. In November 2014, R. finished chemotherapy and entered the next phase of treatments, radiation therapy. Clinically, she had not responded to interventions, and by April 2016, her condition deteriorated. She declined attempts by the association to meet with her or her husband. Meanwhile, she maintained a personal relationship with one anthropologist, a former midwife, who visited her frequently at home, as did the cultural mediator, who lived nearby. At the end of July 2016, her husband called the association to inform them that she had died in her country of origin, where she was seeking additional treatment at the recommendation of family. Neither her husband nor the children were able to accompany her. The husband declined offers of support from the association, such as meetings with a child psychologist for the children, and did not follow up on subsequent calls.

The Case of Mr. S.

Mr. S. arrived in France in 1990. He was originally from a conflict zone in Sri Lanka. He worked there in a bakery but fled the war with the help of family members who had already settled in France. On his way to France, he passed through Germany and Italy, where he still has family. Mr. S. is married to a woman who arrived in France after him, seven years ago. Today, she is the one who takes care of the house, the shopping, and administering her husband's medication. The couple does not have children. Mr. S. suffers from diabetes. He had eye surgery in 2013 and suffered a stroke at the end of 2016. He does not speak French and understands it in a very limited capacity. His wife speaks and understands French somewhat better than he does, but she is more comfortable in English. Mr. S. is under legal guardianship of the state because of his health incapacities.

Paths within the AcSanté Association/Network

The first objective for Mr. S., subsequent to his evaluation, was to arrange access to podiatry care and support for his diabetes. His social benefits supervisor informed his spouse of the possibility of contacting the network AcSanté for help and support. What interested the couple was the podiatry care from which Mr. S. could benefit as part of his treatment for diabetes. His wife came to the association network center and had an interview in English with the coordinator for diabetic healthcare. During this interview she said that her husband drinks a lot and regularly. Accordingly, Mr. S. was eligible for attention from the association because he has diabetes, lives in the 93rd (Seine-Saint-Denis), in a vulnerable situation of social precarity. His Score EPICES was extremely high, precipitating action by association staff to prevent a spiraling social and medical decline. The association obtained consent from Mr. S.'s spouse and from his legal guardian, who had asked the network to take care of him. Mr. S. was not responsive to staff who contacted him. The association then reached out to his primary care physician with a letter explaining what could be envisioned in terms of support. His primary care physician, in turn, conveyed the medical information that he had available. Mr. S. suffered from neuropathy and had suffered a stroke.

He recovered well from the stroke and was mobile, often arriving with one of his friends to help with translating during his medical consultations. Mr. S. also suffered from kidney disease. He had already been hospitalized and, since his return home, his diabetes was becoming unstable. The primary care physician thought that this was due to his diet. Mr. S. met with the association again and this time he agreed to a consultation with a podiatrist. The podiatrist reported that the patient became aggressive at the end of the consultation, that he did not want to settle his account and that he insisted on paying with imitation bankcards.

The association contacted his legal guardian (it took some time before they were able to speak with her) who noted that in order to communicate with Mr. S. she called upon an interpreter who speaks Tamil. The couple had numerous problems: they were in the process of being evicted, they had serious financial difficulties and were heavily in debt. The guardian spoke of psychiatric problems with dangerous behavior (threats made against his wife with a knife, a saber in Mr. S.'s possession with which he threatened her). Because of these stresses, the spouse agreed to seek psychiatric care at the Centre Minkowska (a center where there are ethnopsychologists and psychologists who speak several languages and dialects). However, she quickly abandoned this care. The psychiatrist at Minkowska also wished to see Mr. S., who never showed up for the consultations.

The association set up a home visit with a social worker, the psychologist from the network and the legal guardian as well as a Tamil interpreter. During the visit, Mr. S. spoke from the beginning of the interview with great openness and ease about what he identified as "his problems" (which began around 2001): electrodes that the police from the "European Union" supposedly put under his skin. Each medical intervention, each medical consultation nourished these ideas of devices inserted into his body (through the ears, the anus, the genitals) with the goal of spying on him. He was persuaded that he is also monitored in his home, under surveillance by the police. There is no place where Mr. S. felt safe. Mr. S. indicated that he would kill the police officers who persecute him. He spoke of "forces" that can push him to do things (throw himself on the floor, for example), and he expressed the risk he felt of being able to do harm to himself or others. He described a situation of domestic violence reported by his neighbors and recognized having been violent with his wife. He indicated that it is these problems as well as the transformations provoked in his body by the electrodes that prevent him from working.

Nevertheless, he does not want to stay at home all day; he sometimes goes to a nearby store to buy alcohol. Since he has no money with which to pay, he has debts with the Tamil shopkeepers in the neighborhood. His wife receives insistent demands for reimbursement of her husband's debts. Mr. S. signaled that he goes to the neighborhood police often to complain about his fear of persecution; he also speaks about this with his wife and his primary care physician, but no one believes him. Mr. S. is very open in discussing his symptoms and his suffering tied to these problems. He asks for help. All the same, it seems possible that he feels persecuted by the very people to whom he turns for help (the guardian, the association, as well as unknown and unseen beings). He is not undergoing psychiatric or psychological treatment, and he expressed that he does not want to go to a psychiatric hospital (perhaps because of a previous hospitalization that went poorly).

The association put in place exchanges with the primary care physician to elicit his opinion about Mr. S.'s mental health and the doctor expressed gratitude for the information. He had never noticed his patient's delusional ideas (perhaps because Mr. S.'s friend who accompanied him to consultations did not translate them). The physician had no recommendations for dealing with the situation.

In order to grasp the difficulties in devising possible paths forward for Mr. S., it is necessary to understand that the French "right to health" is complicated and fraught with border crossings for which one requires precise knowledge of the system to understand all of its subtleties. It is necessary to pass by several administrators and interlocutors for a single case. For an individual with Mr. S.'s infirmities, this process is extremely difficult and may ultimately be unsuccessful, even with the multiple interventions attempted by Mr. S.'s guardian, physician, and the AcSanté team. Attempts to assist with legal issues, substance abuse, advanced diabetes, psychotic episodes, and domestic abuse did not, in the long run, lead Mr. S. to a healthy or productive life.

Most people who are eligible to benefit from assistance are those who "accumulate" numerous pejorative social determinants, which means a multiplication of difficulties in accessing health care and social services. Ultimately, when illness combines with precarity, there is likely to be much discouragement for the patient and kin. For the patient, it may seem necessary to fight against the disease and for one's rights simultaneously. Many experience this trajectory as an attack on their dignity as well as an exhausting, fruitless experience.

Conclusion

The Seine-Saint-Denis area exemplifies the intersection of economic and social precarity/polypathology/existential vulnerability, which shape the trajectory for seriously ill patients in need of health care. Immigrants, both documented and undocumented, represent a substantial proportion of the prospective patient pool. In contrast to this substantial patient population, clinicians are in short supply. This region has twelve oncologists for 1.5 million inhabitants, compared to the prestigious Institut Curie cancer center in central Paris, which has thirty oncologists for that facility alone. Multiple social and economic constraints amplify the limitations of the system. As our case studies demonstrate, the existence of a national health system is a necessary but not sufficient condition for assuring health care in the context of "competing priorities." When vital needs such as housing, household revenue, childcare, legal status, are consistently uncertain, sickness becomes merely one intractable problem among others.

The two cases involving gravely ill immigrant patients illustrates this in a concrete way: housing, income, and isolation for one, language and polypathology for another. Therefore, even in a "universal" system, access to care remains an unsolvable problem for the most fragile, and a problem that cannot be resolved by simplistic technocratic solutions. It is in this context that associations external to the hospital itself, such as AcSanté network, claim a mission to evaluate and prioritize patient needs, whether financial, legal, psychological, or social, thus attending to both the physiological, relational, and institutional needs of the patient. As a "network," one objective of AcSanté is to unite the diverse actors relevant to patient needs in a collaborative initiative, designed with each individual patient's particular situation in mind. In the case of Madame R., the network interviewed the patient and family extensively to determine how to prevent further aggravation of precarity in this situation of serious chronic illness. Sargent and anthropological colleagues, as well as an interpreter, phoned, made home visits, and accompanied Madame R. during hospitalizations. Separate from these visits, Madame R. observed that "a woman came [to the house] once a week" from the association, a social worker, on one occasion. Madame R. was not sure why the network followed her case, but she appreciated the support in obtaining AME health insurance, childcare for her youngest child, and assistance with housing. From the point of view of the association, tools such as the Score EPICES served to situate the patient on a scale of precarity and identify particular needs thus far unaddressed. Ultimately, by documenting and resolving issues that limited her ability to attend chemotherapy appointments, the association was one of the primary players in persuading Madame R. to remain in treatment as long as possible.

In the case of Mr. S., the Score EPICES also indicated a high-risk level of precarity. He was financially insolvent, had no form of employment nor was he sufficiently well to work. He had no access to minimum revenue stipends because of his undocumented status and suffered from several illnesses. His untreated diabetes placed him at risk for infections of the limbs, and his delusional episodes posed a risk to himself and others. Unlike Madame R., Mr. S. was resistant to offers of support from the association. His wife briefly attended group psychological consultations at a migrant health care center to which the association referred her, but then withdrew. Mr. S. serves as a reminder that a patient and/or family who refuse legal, economic, and social support or clinical care eventually become outliers in the association network, until such time as circumstances modify their health care choices and perhaps lead them back to AcSanté or a similar organization.

With austerity measures in France reducing hospital budgets, especially for social services, associations external to the hospital take on an even more significant role. The cases we present illustrate the continuing and invaluable role of the associative sector in addressing health precarity, as well as recognizing the borders limiting access to health care and generated by broader economic and structural constraints. Ironically, France is notable for an idealistic national health policy, but for its most vulnerable populations such as immigrants, health care institutions are often only marginally accessible.

Acknowledgments

We gratefully acknowledge the support of the National Science Foundation, NSF BCS1354336, "The Influence of Sociality in Cancer Treatment Decision-Making," PI: Carolyn Sargent. We also thank Kyle Young, Department of Romance Languages and Literatures, for his expert assistance with translation.

Carolyn Sargent is professor of anthropology at Washington University in St. Louis. Her recent interests center on illness and sociality, the transnational production of community, immigration and health, anthropology of cancer, and the politics of reproduction. She has worked in West Africa (Benin, Mali), Jamaica, and her research in progress involves West African and North African immigrants living with breast cancer in France and the collective production of meanings and strategies about this condition.

Professor Laurent Zelek is an oncologist and senologist, Head of the Oncology Department at Hôpital Avicenne in Bobigny, and Professor of Oncology at Université Paris 13 Nord. His research particularly focuses on the role of nutrition and sports in cancer care management and highlights the importance of considering patients' social environment in healthcare provision.

Anne Festa is an independent health consultant. She has worked as a project manager for the French National Institute for Cancer (INCa) and directed several associations in the health sector. Her missions were consistent with making patients actors of their healthcare plan and with reaching out to vulnerable populations at the margins of the system.

Notes

1. Translation from interview by Carolyn Sargent and Martine Beauplet, 21 June 2017. Text slightly modified for purposes of confidentiality.
2. "Emilie Lecroq, Conseillère Départementale de Seine-Saint-Denis, Conseillere." Retrieved 8 January 2022 from www.seinestdenis.fr.

References

Aïach, Pierre. 2010. *Les Inégalités Sociales de Santé: Écrits [The Social Inequalities of Health : Writings]*. Collection *Anthropos*. Paris: Economica.

———. 2013. "La question des Inégalités Sociales de Sante dans un Itinéraire de Chercheur." *Les Tribunes de la Santé* 38: 55–62.

Banki, Susan. 2014. "Precarity of Place: A Complement to the Growing Precariat Literature." *Global Discourse*, (3)3–4: 450–63.

Beauchemin, Chris, Christelle Hamel, and Patrick Simon, eds. 2016. *Trajectoires et Origines. Enquetes sur la Diversite des Populations en France [Trajectories and Origins. Investigations on Population Diversity in France]*. Paris: INED.

Chazan, David. 2018. "Illegal Migrants in Paris Suburb Soar to 400,000 as Hundreds of Migrant Children Sleep on Streets." *The Telegraph*, 5 July.

Cognet, Marguerite. 2014. "Des Inégalités d'Accès aux Soins aux Discriminations en Santé [From Heathcare Access Inequalities to Health Discrimination]." *Rhizome* 52 (June): 8.

Fassin, Didier. 2004. "Social Illegitimacy as a Foundation of Health Inequality: How the Political Treatment of Immigrants Illuminates a French Paradox." In *Unhealthy Health Policy*, ed. Arachu Castro and Merill Singer, 203–14. Lanham, MD: Rowman and Littlefield.

Fourmy, Sebastian. 2013. *The True Cost of Austerity and Inequality in France: A Case Study*. Oxford: Oxfam International.

INCa (Institut National du Cancer). 2014. *Plan Cancer 2009–2013*. Retrieved 3 September 2014 https://www.e-cancer.fr/Institut-national-du-cancer/Strategie-de-lutte-contre-les-cancers-en-France.

Insée (Institut National de la Statistique et des Etudes Economiques). 2011. *Populations légales 2011–93-Seine-Saint-Denis: Recensement de la Population 2011- Limites Territoriales au 1er janvier 2013 [Legal Populations 2011-93-Seine-St-Denis : 2011 Population Census – Territorial Limits on January 1st, 2013]*. Paris: INSEE.

Jaouen, Arthur. 2015. *Analyse des Leviers d'Amélioration/d'Aggravation dans le Suivi de Femmes Atteintes de Cancer du Sein en Situation de Précarité, Prises en Charge par le Réseau AcSanté 93, en Seine-Saint-Denis [Analysis of Improvement/Deterioration Factors for Poor Women with Breast Cancer, Followed by the AcSanté 93 Network, in Seine-Saint-Denis]*. Paris: Université de Versailles.

Larchanché, Stéphanie. 2012. "Intangible Obstacles: Health Implications of Stigmatization, Structural Violence, and Fear among Undocumented Immigrants in France." *Social Science and Medicine* 74: 858–63.

Sargent, Carolyn, and Laurence Kotobi. 2017. "Austerity and Its Implications for Immigrant Health in France." *Social Science and Medicine* 187: 259–67.

Sass, Catherine, Jean-Jacques Moulin, René Guéguen, Loïc Abric, Virginie Dauphinot, Caroline Dupré, Jean Pierre Giordanella, Florence Girard, Catherine Guenot, Émilie Labbe, Emilio La Rosa, Pierre Magnier, Édith Martin, Bernard Royer, Michèle Rubirola, and Laurent Gerbaud. "Le Score Epices: un Score Individuel de Précarité. Construction du Score et Mesures des Relations avec des Données de Santé, dans une Population de 197,389 Personnes [The EPICES Score : A Person-Based Score Measuring Precarity. Elaboration of the Score and Examination of Relations with Health Data, for a Population of 197,389]." *Bulletin Epidemiologie Hebdomadaire* 14: 92–95.

Simonet, Daniel. 2013. "New Public Management and the Reform of French Public Hospitals." *Journal of Public Affaires* 13 (3): 260–71.

Standing, Guy. 2011. *The Precariat.* London: Bloomsbury Academic.

Stuckler, David, and Sanjay Basu. 2013. *The Body Economic: Why Austerity Kills: Recessions, Budget Battles, and the Politics of Life and Death.* New York: Basic Books.

Torsoli, Albertina. 2013. "France's Health-Care System Is Going Broke." *Bloomberg Business Week.* Retrieved 9 September 2016 from https://www.bloomberg.com/news/articles/2013–01–03/frances-healthcare-system-is-going-broke.

Zelek, Laurent, Chloe Bodere, Delphine Bourlier, and Anne Festa. 2015. "Enhancing Compliance with National Nutrition Recommendations in Breast Cancer Survivors. Experience in an Underprivileged Community." *Cancer Research* 75(9): 1–11.

6
Doctors Challenging Borders
The Successes and Dilemmas of Syrian-American Medical Humanitarians

Rania Kassab Sweis

One day during a medical workshop held by a global humanitarian organization I hereafter call Medical Relief for Syria (MRS), Mohamad, a humanitarian doctor, talked to me about the devastating emotional effects the ongoing Syrian Civil War has had on him.[1] While sitting in a lounge chair outside a coffee shop in Washington, DC, he extended his right arm out as far as it could go with the wrist facing up, as if he were about to give blood. "Look," he pleaded, "I'm emotionally drained from this war. If someone were to cut me right here right now, nothing would come out." Mohamad kept referring to a metaphoric draining of his own body, a sense of personal and professional depletion brought on by his routine witnessing of bodily violence and countless deaths since the Syrian crisis-turned-civil-war began. Later in our conversation, he went on to explain a sense of shared suffering he believed the doctors of this organization experienced collectively, as US immigrants who have lived in, grown up, and studied in Syria, and who are now witnessing the war both from afar and through the suffering of their patients during global medical missions. "We're all feeling helpless," he softly commented in recalling this dislocation in war, "helpless and hopeless." For Mohamad, this personal attachment and sense of hopeless depletion—the emptiness as he suggested by using the metaphor of draining blood—stemmed from a unique cultural location he and other MRS doctors occupied within the structures of global humanitarianism: they were neither detached in terms of national affiliation, nor local and living within the society receiving aid. How are we to situate Mohamad's experiences within humanitarianism when global aid work is typically imagined through a singular and hegemonic East/West or North/South divide? How does Mohamad, and other MRS doctors, challenge conventional notions of who gives global aid?

In many ways, Mohamad unsettles many of the assumptions present in public discourse and scholarship about who travels across national borders to intervene to provide life-saving medical aid to vulnerable populations in the Global South. As Adia Benton observes, it is white Americans and Europeans that dominate global health and humanitarian industries and whose experiences and narratives feature prominently in public discourse and scholarship about global aid.[2] In contrast to those prominent experiences and narratives, and by drawing on the lives and motivations of MRS doctors like Mohamad, I offer in this chapter an alternative framework through which we can think about global medical aid workers. In short, I capture some of the successes, dilemmas, and embodied experiences of MRS doctors who, as Muslim and Arab global aid workers, do not resemble the dominant figures, the cultural prototype, through which global aid is practiced. As Nadia El-Shaarawi and Stéphanie Larchanché note in the introduction of this edited volume, migrants are sometimes cast as outsiders and as suspicious, threatening subjects due to nationalistic and xenophobic policies and rhetoric. As such they face countless obstacles, including racism and stigma. I will demonstrate in this chapter how, amid an increasingly Islamophobic global landscape, MRS doctors experience some of these same challenges in their attempt to provide care to extremely vulnerable Syrians. In doing so, I want to encourage more nuanced and in-depth analyses of the various racial and cultural hierarchies that exist within global humanitarianism for aid workers.

By shifting my ethnographic focus away from aid recipients, who are the most vulnerable subjects in the Syrian Civil War, to the providers of aid, I join other scholars of humanitarianism who have recently begun to foreground the professional lives and situated practices of global aid workers in their research.[3] These scholars have rightfully shown that ethnographic explorations into the identities, obligations, and attachments of aid workers is critical if we are to grasp the full scale of how humanitarianism operates in the world today, both as human practice and as a mechanism of contemporary global governance.[4] By shining an ethnographic light on aid workers, these works have beautifully and forcefully captured the "dual direction" (Bornstein 2005; Hunleth 2017) of global humanitarian encounters—in other words, how both the givers and receivers of aid are observably and ritualistically transformed through humanitarian action.

Since the start of Syrian popular uprisings turned Civil War (2011–present), the Syrian-American doctors of MRS have been at the forefront of the violence, delivering much-needed emergency care to wounded and suffering Syrians. They volunteer time, resources, and medical expertise in a network of elaborate makeshift clinics and informal field hospitals, both inside Syria and in surrounding Jordanian, Turkish, and Lebanese refugee camps. Sometimes the very first responders to aerial bombardment, they routinely risk their lives working in besieged areas or in conditions of extreme crisis. Moreover, precisely because of their widespread life-saving potential, and despite international laws condemning attacks on medical personnel in war zones, they are often the objects of militarized violence themselves. As a consortium of aid organizations have repeatedly asserted since the start of the Syrian crisis, the bombing of medical facilities inside Syria and the targeting of medical personnel are not byproducts of the violence. Rather they are a defining feature of the Syrian Civil War.[5] With roughly half a million fatalities to date and nearly half of Syria's prewar population of 21 million people either internally or external displaced, the Syrian Civil War has precipitated what the UN and scholars are calling the world's worse humanitarian upheaval since World War II (Pearlman 2017). Local doctors and Arab emigrants, not foreign doctors, continue to provide the majority of life-saving aid to suffering Syrians in and around Syria. And yet, as a social category with remarkable outcomes for those experiencing the violence of war firsthand, they remain underrepresented in social science scholarship.

The research in this chapter is based on intermittent interviews and observations I conducted in the United States with MRS doctors between 2014 and 2018. As a global organization dedicated to medical relief, MRS stands out as culturally "Syrian." Nearly all of its members are Syrian immigrants living and working in Europe or the United States. Their age ranges span from early thirties to mid-sixties, and because the majority of doctors conducting international medical missions are men, the voices captured in this research are unequally those of men. However, women doctors, nurses, and healthcare administrators continue to participate in meaningful, ongoing aid work with MRS, although in relatively lesser numbers. Claiming to work on the frontlines of war, the organization's initial aims were to service vulnerable Syrians who lacked access to emergency or long-term healthcare due to the ongoing political violence. But in recent years, as its successes amid the Syrian war grew, it sought to branch out and care for other vulnerable, poor, or displaced populations in countries such as Egypt or Greece. The majority of MRS's funding comes from the US, French, and German governments, but a significant portion also stems from fundraising efforts targeting private donors and its own organization members as well. As an organization with hundreds of participating doctors and dozens of "chapters" situated across the United States and the UK, MRS unsettles the imaginary East/West divide through which much global aid work is believed to travel. Its members view themselves as global experts wavering between East and West; their bilingual fluency in both Arabic and English speaks most directly to this status. In addition, they are motivated by discourses other than the desire to relinquish a life of material wealth and excess (Redfield 2013), the hope of remedying deep-seated isolation and loneliness (Malkki 2015), or the goal of assisting distant, racialized sufferers in far way places (Fassin 2001). As I carried out this research with MRS doctors during their medical workshops or professional conferences, I strove to capture their specific aid-based aspirations and cultural discourses. In doing so, I approached humanitarianism ethnographically and not as an absolute. That is, I traced it "as an array of particular embodied, situated practices emanating from the humanitarian desire to alleviate the suffering of others" (Redfield 2005: 330).

Following Didier Fassin's seminal work on the inherent inequalities shaping global humanitarian politics today, my findings suggest that MRS doctors are positioned precariously with a global "hierarchy of humanitarians" that deems, as Fassin noted in tracing various asymmetries between different kinds of aid workers, some lives less worthy of mobility and protection than others. To this end, scholars of humanitarianism have only recently begun to move away from a focus on foreign American or European global aid workers in their studies, centering their questions instead on the identities and predicaments of local aid workers in the Global South (Fassin and Rechtman 2009; Omidian and Panter-Brick 2015). While these voices remain critically underrepresented in our work and warrant further attention, I contend that MRS doctors experience a unique set of predicaments and successes, all of which owe to their status as immigrant foreign aid workers who are liminally positioned between "local" and "foreign" aid workers and who retain both personal and professional attachments to the society receiving aid. This ambiguous location, neither inside nor outside of the society receiving aid, requires its own line of scholarly interrogation, as it can help us grasp some of the complex yet often overlooked nuances that exist between global aid workers and within large-scale humanitarian institutions today. Let me turn to my fieldwork with MRS to help crystalize my point about a hierarchy of global humanitarians.

Ambiguous Locations: Wavering between Cultural Attachment and Professional Expertise

Several interrelated themes emerged from my interviews with MRS doctors after I asked how they saw themselves as Syrian-Americans and as global aid workers in the context of the Syrian war. Here, I will discuss two of the most prominent themes because they played a central role in the doctors' narratives. The first theme was that of cultural attachment, which was typically articulated as a love of homeland or sense of national belonging. Here, doctors attempted to re-establish themselves as good Syrian subjects. The second theme was that of professional expertise and solidarity, echoing much of Liisa Malkki's findings in a masterful study of Finnish Red Cross workers who provide global aid (2015). Malkki contends that professional dispositions should be thought of structurally—in terms of "ideals" that work for a particular group of aid workers and situate them socially. For MRS doctors, these ideals reinforced their status as experts and consisted of universalized knowledge, including medical neutrality and standardized training. While reinforcing each other at times, or overlapping, these two broad themes appeared distinct in the doctors' responses. Below I provide several notable interview accounts that either bound together or differentiated these ideas for the doctors. Taken together, the insights demonstrate how MRS doctors saw themselves as occupying an ambiguous, at times disadvantaged, position, while at other times they remained privileged givers of care within a global hierarchy of humanitarians.

Cultural Attachment

In the first theme of cultural attachment, doctors emphasized their shared Syrian heritage, cultural identities, or enduring love of "homeland" in global aid work. Additionally, when it came to the subject of transnational mobility, they appeared as subjects who were "bound to place" (Brown 2006) in a manner unlike white American and European global aid workers, but also as subjects who have had to navigate exclusionary politics due to their specific national, racial, or cultural associations. For instance, during one organization meeting in 2017, where the subject of medical neutrality in global aid work was being discussed, an MRS doctor stood up and raised a concern about his embattled process of crossing borders both before and after his global aid missions. He complained about President Trump's (then recent) travel ban on seven Muslim majority countries, for which Syria was one. In a pleading, yet deviant tone, he addressed his audience:

> Why can't they make it easier for us doctors to travel to provide this help? What can we do to get immunity from these policies so we can do our duties? We are completely exposed and vulnerable to this legislation and no one is supporting us. Some even call us terrorists!

In this comment, we get a glimpse of how aid can engender a sense of vulnerability and precarity for doctors, particularly when faced with discriminatory border policies. Shortly thereafter, another doctor in the meeting stood up and echoed this concern, mentioning that at present, the majority of British (read western European) medical students embark on some kind of global medical mission without proper experience or extensive training in emergency medical relief—the kind of skills, he suggested, MRS doctors possess—yet also without experiencing the same exclusionary policies when traveling, including humiliating border interrogations. "Those doctors," he pointed out to the group, "are not questioned and are not viewed as problems or threats." Doctors in the audience nodded vigorously in agreement as he went on to explain that such policies are obstacles to organizational success; in other words, they work to prevent MRS doctors from conducting the swiftest, most efficient, life-saving aid work possible.

Many of the MRS doctors I interviewed also shared with me how their love of homeland and deep sense of belonging to Syria shaped their subjectivities and practices as aid givers. They emphasized their cultural knowledge of the place undergoing crisis, a collective Syrian-ness in some respects, and often this propelled them into choosing global aid work in the first place. And this sense of belonging to the society receiving aid undergirded their ongoing professional commitments to global aid work in the context of the war. For example, Ibrahim, another MRS doctor, discussed with me why he chose to join MRS's medical missions when the war first broke out. He spoke about feeling "close" to the recipient population culturally, and even described the sentiment of feeling "warmth" during the medical humanitarian encounter. For him, warmth meant more than simple proximity to his aid recipients. It implied a kind of cultural adequacy, which he believed only Syrian doctors with intimate histories and cultural knowledge about life in Syria possess. As he explained:

> Syrian doctors and the Syrian population are very close. We have not been born with a silver spoon in our mouths. Maybe this factor makes us more

> humble. It's easier for us to go there and be accepted, we sit on floors, eat off of one plate with our hands, we show emotional warmth.

Here, Ibrahim also juxtaposed doctors like himself with other, presumably white and foreign, aid workers whom he suggests are more privileged than him, having been born with "silver spoons" in their mouths. As a result of this hierarchal distinction in aid work, he believed "other" doctors lacked the cultural knowledge necessary to be similarly "close" to Syrian aid recipients during this war.

Majed shared a similar sentiment when I asked him why he joined MRS medical missions and embarked on global aid work. In his response, however, he highlighted the love he felt for both country and population, as he explained: "When you love your country, you love your people, and when you see our people being killed, even though it's by your people, you just can't help but help those who need it."

In my interviews with other MRS doctors, the subject of cultural attachment and a feeling of belonging to the society receiving aid surfaced through the metaphor of a debt repayment, where doctors expressed loyalty to a nation (Syria) and the desire to "give back" to Syria through medical aid because they believed they owed the place or its people a service. For example, here is how Wael put it when discussing why he participated in MRS medical missions:

> I do this work because I have a sense of debt to repay. My education was practically free in Syria. Here, I see medical students pay hundreds of thousands of dollars for their education. I feel I have to pay this back by helping [Syria]. I feel I have to do something.

Other doctors had more complex feelings of national belonging, owing to their status as naturalized American citizens who grew up in Syria. Mohamad, whom I mentioned at the start of this chapter, had this to say in discussing why he engaged in aid work with MRS. He emphasized dual intersecting "feelings" of nationhood and an enduring love for the "Syrian people," which drove his global aid commitments. As he explained:

> The United States is my home. I love it here. This country gave me opportunities, and it is my home country. This country gave me everything. I care about my friends, family, the places I went to [in Syria]. And I am loyal to the Syrian people. I still love Syria, and I still love the Syrian people. And I feel sorry for them. I do whatever I can to help them because of this feeling.

Like many other MRS doctors, Mohamad immigrated to the United States in his early twenties after completing basic medical training in Syria. He was middle-aged when I met him and expressed great pride in his own professional success, having grown a thriving private practice in nephrology. In the statement above, he notes having multiple national attachments connected to his aid work, a national affiliation (as a naturalized American citizen) operating alongside an enduring love of Syria. Despite his loyalty to "the Syrian people," he considers only one place his "home"—

the United States. Having these specific identity markers—Syrian, American, professional, and aid worker—situates him differently, from both local aid workers in Syria, and white American or European aid workers who are assumed to operate transnationally as universal, detached, or culture-free actors.

Professional Expertise

MRS doctors also commented on the centrality of their professional commitments to advancing global aid work, as well as their status as highly trained, transnational experts who continually strive to improve humanitarianism by increasing successful outcomes for their recipients. In these narratives, doctors stressed how a set of professional ethics guided their humanitarian practices, one of which was the concept of medical neutrality in times of war. As practicing physicians, they strove to uphold an ethic of saving universal human life in its barest and most basic form, or, as Miriam Ticktin (2011) observed, they legitimated biological life in their humanitarian discourses—life devoid of politics, culture, and history. Drawing on the work of philosopher Georgio Agamben, Peter Redfield termed this medical humanitarian ethic a "minimalist biopolitics," one that reflects the basic value of life for which humanitarians seek to defend (2005: 329–30). In many of the responses I received, MRS doctors invoked the figure of the dreaded "soldier" to reinforce their ethic of minimalist biopolitics. As subjects who have lived in Syria under what they described as a brutal authoritarian regime, the soldier often constituted the embodiment of state militarized violence. They asserted that even when faced with this representational figure in aid, their professional impulse for saving human life through medical action would not be disturbed. As Ibrahim elucidated:

> We are in the business of saving lives, and we save lives. As doctors, we treat even soldiers without question. We are not equipped to decide who is friend or enemy. We work on saving lives and this is a universal attitude. Human life is human life.

Similarly, Majed, another MRS doctor, reiterated his commitments to professionalism by privileging medical "training" before political or national attachment. In his narrative, he too invoked the figure of the soldier to represent state violence and governmental illegitimacy. As he put it:

> I was trained to help whoever needs the help. Even the soldier. I'm not a lawyer or a judge. I don't do legal work. I have an obligation to help people, first as physician, and second, as a national of my country.

As we can see in Majed's articulation, the preservation of universalized human life and the maintenance of physical existence—even with respect to the soldier—is of paramount importance, it remains on a higher threshold of value when compared to other commitments. For him, one comes "first" (saving human life) while the other is "second" (national attachment). Ibrahim also explained how he navigated the two competing realms of professionalism and politics, but rather than describe the distinction in terms of one coming before the other, as Majed did in the quote above, he used the metaphor of a white doctor's coat. For Ibrahim, his white coat signified a critical transition in identity—movement from politically engaged citizen-subject to practicing physician charged with upholding universalized medical ethics. He asserted:

> When I am a doctor, I am a doctor. When I take off my coat and just wear my clothes, I can conduct my civic duty. Now, if I have a political agenda or make a political statement, I cannot be a doctor, so I do not wear my coat. You cannot have a conflict of interest and let your political views dictate you [as a doctor]. That is against our profession.

As these narratives indicate, MRS doctors strove to uphold an ethic of medical professionalism and impartiality in their work. Such an ethic stipulated that the saving of universal human life, life in its barest biological form, remained the ultimate aim of MRS medical humanitarian action. MRS doctors articulated this goal by drawing clear distinctions between their civic and professional duties and between their political and medical attachments. For them, the distinctions between politics and medicine were critical, as they provided clear markers for success in global aid work while situating each doctor within a broader network of global professionals charged with upholding recipient biological integrity. Here, as for medical humanitarians elsewhere, the discourse of apolitical humanitarian action, driven by the legitimacy of universalized human life, framed the doctors' responses.

Another manner by which MRS doctors reinforced their sense of professional solidary with each other was through the continuous refinement of their medical humanitarian expertise. They engaged in intensive pedagogical sessions during meetings or workshops, where they shared case studies from previous missions and advised each other on best humanitarian practices. During such sessions, MRS doctors gathered in professional settings and shared a collective impulse to do "better medicine." This entailed improving technical, medical skills in the field when faced with a lack of infrastructure, such as emergency surgeries in the aftermath of aerial bombardment or the treatment of dialysis patients in ill-equipped refugee camps. In these professional conversations, doctors re-established themselves as the ideal experts most capable to provide aid to suffering Syrians. They often drew on their privileged status as highly trained medical professionals armed with vast resources and expert knowledge to assert these claims. They also strove to cultivate new and innovative skills that would be applied transnationally and attuned to the context of the violence in Syria. For MRS doctors, enhancing technical capabilities was an important avenue through which they could increase successful recipient outcomes and reduce human suffering. These aspects of doing better, more efficient humanitarian work all refracted back onto what it meant to be a good Syrian subject and exemplary humanitarian doctor during this particular war.

For Ibrahim, the discourse of professional expertise was closely connected to a desire to return to Syria and rebuild a war-torn landscape. Having grown a successful practice in the United States after immigrating decades ago upon completing basic medical training in Syria, he viewed himself as now properly equipped with the knowledge and resources necessary to accomplish national rebuilding. Like other

MRS doctors, he spoke of this desire to rebuild in terms of a duty, referencing his privileged status vis-à-vis Syrians who are in the country, unable to emigrate, and experiencing the violence firsthand. For Ibrahim, rebuilding would help level global inequalities that exist between MRS doctors and Syrians suffering the war. For instance, in discussing expert knowledge of MRS members, he commented:

> We are all at the peak of our professional performance, and now we are ready to start making plans to go back to Syria. We left Syria knowing we would seek better economic opportunity, more education, we were going to build a new life in the land behind the oceans and the seas. And we knew we might come back sometime. But now we are asking, "when is it going to be safe to go back?" I'm willing to go and train students, technicians, nurses, and treat patients for free. I don't need the luxury that I imagined twenty years ago. We are physicians who are now waiting for it to be safe enough so we can start going back to rebuild, in any shape or form.

In this quote, Ibrahim situates MRS doctors as ideal experts, at the "peak" of their careers, who are ready to help in the process of postwar national rebuilding. Armed with adequate professional skills, he viewed himself as engaging, one day, in medical pedagogy, which entailed training local healthcare professionals in more advanced medicine. In this way, MRS doctors, like other global medical humanitarians, understand themselves as powerful, resource-rich givers of aid when it comes to their recipients. And yet, due to their immigrant status, cultural attachments, and Muslim identities, they are situated on a somewhat "lower rung" (Benton 2016) withn a global hierarchy of humanitarians when compared to their American and European counterparts. These multiple and intersecting factors, wavering between privilege and vulnerability, contribute to the ambiguous location MRS doctors find themselves in within global aid.

Concluding Thoughts

In writing about the doctors working for the French-based medical humanitarian organization Médecins Sans Frontières, Peter Redfield contends that identities matter when it comes to global aid work. This means that the one who has access to a border-free world, and the one who does not, shapes the political contours and cultural makeup of global humanitarian landscapes. Indeed, identities have material and social effects. As I have shown in this article, for MRS, these effects are significant within the humanitarian giver and recipient relationship, but they are also significant with respect to a set of social and racial hierarchies that exist between global medical humanitarians—the givers of aid. As a case study, MRS doctors who continue to provide life-saving aid to Syrian victims of war help solidify these points about identity in aid work. As distant observers and entrenched experts in the Syrian Civil War, they consider themselves vulnerable yet powerful subjects. The narratives captured in this chapter speak to their multidimensional needs, obligations, and desires, as well as to challenges connected to their immigrant, Muslim status. They have had to navigate multiple cultural worlds, in much the same way many of the migrant subjects whose experiences animate this edited volume. Yet as medical providers, they understand their work as situated between a set of interrelated situations that waver between cultural affiliation and professional attachment. For them, global aid work signifies a professional impulse to save universal human (biological) life in its barest, most basic form. But for them aid work is also much more than that. It reflects a continuous refinement of medical expertise and means toward professional solidarity with other Syrian doctors. In addition, it involves a love of national homeland(s) and a longing for return and rebuilding in war-ravaged Syria. Since the start of the Syrian crisis, doctors like Mohamad, Ibrahim, Wael, and Majed have faced a set of unique physical and emotional challenges that owe to their complex cultural identities, from Islamophobic border policies that mark them as potential threats or even "terrorists" to the emotional consequences brought on by witnessing death and destruction in Syria from afar and through their suffering patients. As Mohamad illustrated best at the start of this chapter, MRS doctors grapple with these intimate sentiments, these consequences of war, and with a literal and metaphoric "wound that bleeds" (see Introduction to this volume).

At the time of this writing, the violence and destruction in Syria persists. As global medical aid becomes more of a permanent fixture there, and in crisis zones throughout the region, understanding each side of the global medical humanitarian encounter—between aid givers and receivers on the one hand, and global aid workers who are hierarchically situated on the other—provides new insights into the nature of violence in the region and its effects on human lives. War as we have long observed has lasting, pernicious effects upon bodies, populations, and infrastructures.[6] As humanitarian institutions come to fill in the gaps left open by devastated healthcare structures, as is the case inside Syria and in surrounding refugee camps, humanitarian workers have increasingly emerged as the sole healthcare providers to vulnerable populations. Turning attention to their "reasonings" (Fassin 2012), including their politics, desires, and dilemmas, alongside those of aid recipients allows for a better reckoning of humanitarian government as human practice.

Rania Kassab Sweis is associate professor of anthropology at the University of Richmond. Her research interests center on critical medical anthropology, global health and medical humanitarianism, transnational feminist theory, and the Middle East and North Africa region. Her first book project, titled *Paradoxes of Care: Children and Global Medical Aid in Egypt*, (Stanford University Press, 2021) is based on more than two years of in-depth fieldwork in Cairo and a southern Egyptian village. It traces the experiences and everyday lives of vulnerable children who receive global medical assistance. Her second book project focuses on the politics of medical humanitarianism in the Syrian Civil War, with a focus on the lives and practices of local doctors and emergency healthcare workers.

Acknowledgments

The research upon which this chapter is based was supported by a series of generous grants from the University of Richmond. Portions of this chapter appeared in the article by Sweis, "Doctors with Borders: Hierarchies of Humanitarians and the Syrian Civil War." *The International Journal of Middle East Studies* 51 (2019).

Notes

1. All of the names of people and key organizations in this research have been changed in order to protect the identities of human subjects in line with Institutional Review Board protocols.
2. See especially the work of Adia Benton (2016) on race and when it comes to African expatriates who work in global aid industries.
3. Some recent works on this subject include Benton (2016); Fassin (2012); Hamdy and Bayoumi (2016); Malkki (2015); Naguib (2017); Redfield (2013).
4. See Sweis (2012, 2017a, 2017b).
5. From the UN Security Council Resolution 2286 (2016) and "The Failure of UN Security Council Resolution 2286 in Preventing Attacks on Healthcare in Syria," Syrian-American Medical Society, January 2017, Press Release.
6. See especially De Rond (2016); Ticktin (2011).

References

Benton, Adia. 2016. "African Expatriates and Race in the Anthropology of Humanitarianism." *Critical African Studies* 8(3): 266–77. https://doi.org/10.1080/21681392.2016.1244956.

Bornstein, Erica. 2005. *The Spirit of Development: Protestant NGOs, Morality, and Economics in Zimbabwe*. Stanford, CA: Stanford University Press.

Brown, Wendy. 2006. *Regulating Aversion: Tolerance in the Age of Identity and Empire*. Princeton, NJ: Princeton University Press.

De Rond, Mark. 2017. *Doctors at War: Life and Death in a Field Hospital*. Ithaca: Cornell University Press.

Fassin, Didier. 2001. "The Biopolitics of Otherness: Undocumented Foreigners and Racial Discrimination in French Public Debate." *Anthropology Today* 17(1): 3–7.

———. 2012. *Humanitarian Reason: A Moral History of the Present*. Berkeley: University of California Press.

Fassin, Didier, and Richard Rechtman. 2009. *The Empire of Trauma: An Inquiry into the Condition of Victimhood*. Princeton, NJ: Princeton University Press.

Hamdy, Sherine F., and Soha Bayoumi. 2016. "Egypt's Popular Uprising and the Stakes of Medical Neutrality." *Culture, Medicine, and Psychiatry*. http://doi.org/10.1007/s11013-015-9468-1.

Hunleth, Jean. 2017. *Children as Caregivers: The Global Fight against Tuberculosis and HIV in Zambia*. New Brunswick, NJ: Rutgers University Press.

Malkki, Liisa H. 2015. *The Need to Help: The Domestic Arts of International Humanitarianism*. Durham, NC: Duke University Press.

Naguib, Nefissa. 2017. "Middle East Encounters 69 Degrees North Latitude: Syrian Refugees and Everyday Humanitarianism in the Arctic." *International Journal of Middle East Studies* 49: 645–60.

Omidian, Patricia, and Catherine Panter-Brick. 2015. "Dignity under Extreme Duress: The Moral and Emotional Landscape of Local Humanitarian Workers in the Afghan-Pakistan Border Areas." In *Medical Humanitarianism: Ethnographies of Practice*, ed. Sharon Abramowitz and Catherine Panter-Brick, 23–40. Philadelphia: University of Pennsylvania Press.

Pearlman, Wendy. 2017. *We Crossed a Bridge and it Trembled: Voices from Syria*. New York: HarperCollins.

Redfield, Peter. 2005. "Doctors, Borders, and Life in Crisis." *Cultural Anthropology* 20(3): 328–61.

———. 2013. *Life in Crisis: The Ethical Journey of Doctors without Borders*. Berkeley: University of California Press.

Sweis, Rania Kassab. 2012. "Saving Egypt's Village Girls: Rights, Embodiment and Gendered Vulnerability in a Global Youth Initiative." *Journal of Middle East Women's Studies* 8(2): 26–50.

———. 2017a. "Children as Biological Sufferers? The Paradox of International Medical Aid for Homeless Children in Cairo." *Childhood* 24(4): 502–16.

———. 2017b. "Security and the Traumatized Street Child: How Gender Shapes International Psychiatric Aid in Cairo." *Medical Anthropology Quarterly* 32(1): 5–21.

———. 2019. "Doctors with Borders: Hierarchies of Humanitarians and the Syrian Civil War." *International Journal of Middle East Studies* 51(4): 587–601. http://doi.org/10.1017/s0020743819000643.

Ticktin, Miriam. 2011. *Casualties of Care: Immigration and the Politics of Humanitarianism in France*. Berkeley, Los Angeles, London: University of California Press.

PART III

Challenging Policy Borders

Migration policies are central mechanisms that define and enforce borders by directly limiting human mobility and agency. Beyond the policies that create, maintain, and police nation-state and other territorial and political borders, a range of policies can be understood as performing bordering to the extent that they classify and exclude groups of people. In this section, we turn to the direct and indirect health effects of migration policy. The contributions in this section challenge us to broaden our understanding of the relations between health and policy in the realm of migration, moving beyond a narrow focus on health policy to consider how migration and border policy, broadly construed, affects the health and well-being of individuals and communities. They also urge us to consider the economic and political interests that undergird such policies. While both chapters in this section draw on ethnographic work in the United States, the politics and policies they describe, including detention, separation, and the construction of migrants as a "burden," have both been inspired by, and in turn inspired, similar policies in other countries. In any case, the themes of increasingly restrictive migration policies and their effects on migrants will resonate in a wide range of contemporary contexts.

This section asks:

What are the explicit and implicit politics of migration policies? What underlying assumptions and rhetorics do they draw on, and what alternative agendas do they serve? How do such policies affect migrants' health and well-being? How, and on what grounds, can migrants contest such policies?

Chapter 7 unveils the underlying political and financial stakes of restrictive migration policies that enshrine and formalize a "public charge" rhetoric. This term rests on a narrative of racialization that is particularly rooted in the United States but will be familiar in other contexts where migrants are scapegoated as a burden, especially on healthcare, education, and welfare systems. This chapter revisits notions introduced in the first section of this volume, namely moral hierarchies of deservingness and belonging, that serve to restrict certain migrants' access to legal status and related benefits such as food or healthcare assistance. It also critiques abusive and traumatizing detention conditions for undocumented migrants at the border, as well as drawing attention to how explicitly punitive policies, such as the strategic use of family separation, have long-lasting mental health consequences.

Chapter 8 offers us the opportunity to consider how migrants challenge both how punitive and denigrating policies represent them in addition to disputing the policies themselves. As migrants are often denied access to the rights, responsibilities, and recognition associated with citizenship, how can they make their political demands and needs heard? One possible answer that this chapter offers is an encouragement to think of the possibilities for political action at different scales. In the chapter, migrants, facing xenophobic migration policy at the federal level, seek to assert their agency and voices as political subjects at the state level instead. Through such actions, they are able to make policy-related violence and its health consequences visible and demand formal acknowledgement of their rights.

7
Citizenship for Sale and Legality Foreclosed
Immigration, Financialization, and the US Health Care System

Nolan Kline

On an international flight returning to the United States from a professional meeting in 2019, I chatted with a passenger next to me from Canada. He was in his thirties, and as part of our small talk, we discussed significant others, nightlife in the German city we were departing, and our professions. When the passenger asked me what I did for a living, I told him I was a professor of anthropology; eventually, he asked what kind of research I did. As Nadia El-Shaarawi and Stéphanie Larchanché describe in the introduction to this volume, migration is one of the most polarizing issues of our time, and as someone who studies migration and health, I often hesitate to tell people much about my work. I decided to tell my seatmate about my work, though, since some of my research focused on anti-immigrant sentiment following the election of Donald Trump as US president, and I was curious to know how my seat companion for the next eight hours might react to my research. Curiously, he replied by saying "oh, you kind of do the opposite of what I do." Intrigued, I asked him about his profession, and he informed me he was a consultant and citizenship broker. "I work with wealthy clients to find them investments that will earn them citizenship in another country," he said. Since we had been talking about politics, including how some progressive voters in the United States wished Canadian Prime Minister Justin Trudeau were US President, he noted the US market for his work had increased following Trump's election. "There are a lot of wealthy people in the US who are freaked out by Trump, so they're trying to find a place where they can easily get dual citizenship. I find an investment for them and my job is to make all that happen for them as seamlessly as possible. Sometimes I go buy property for clients and handle all of it for them." Comparing our work and the populations we work with, the passenger next to me added, "it seems like we work on the same issue but with opposite populations: you're looking at people trying to get into a country to escape poverty, and I'm working with people trying to escape their country by using their money to buy themselves citizenship somewhere else."

As the passenger next to me suggested, there is a global market for what the financial industry refers to as "citizenship investments" or "immigrant investor programs." Simultaneously, there are numerous transnational migration movements and related economic, political, and social insecurities that have resulted in efforts to exclude migrants from entering the same nations that offer authorized immigration status through investment. In this chapter, I examine the United States' role in excluding immigrants based on conflated economic and health concerns, rooted in racially informed ideology. I specifically examine two policy contexts: first, I consider immigration exclusions related to concerns about immigrants being "a public charge," or burdening the public financially. Public charge concerns have become a rhetorical element of an overall aggressive approach to immigration enforcement in the United States, and public charge anxieties reinforce notions of undocumented immigrants being perceived as drains on the overall US health care system. Second, I consider a visa policy that expedites authorized immigration statuses to immigrants who invest large sums of money in the United States, situating the policy in a global context.

In focusing on these policies, I consider how both the US healthcare and immigration systems have become increasingly financialized. I further examine how immigration regimes that punish immigrants with precarious legal statuses produce revenue for private corporations and simultaneously promote nativist notions of belonging that conflate race, health, and belonging. Situating these policies in the US political context, I describe how the Trump administration both doubled-down on aggressive enforcement regimes and problematically advertised citizenship investment programs. Overall, I show how these simultaneous actions demonstrate how rights and entitlements themselves are transformed into commodities, demanding policy attention.

No Entry: Race, Health, and Public Charge Paranoia in the United States

As Sarah Willen and Jennifer Cook (this volume) show, public charge rhetoric shaped governmental policy agendas and political talking points during the Trump administration, as demonstrated by acting director of the United States Citizenship and Immigration Service Ken Cuccinelli suggesting only immigrants who can "stand on their own two feet" should be permitted into the country. Long before the Trump administration, however, the United States conflated immigration policy, health status, and economics. For example, immigration authorities in the early twentieth century denied immigrants entry into the country based on concerns of immigrants being a "public charge:" a financial burden to the broader public based on not being able to take care of one's self due to poor health or other circumstances (Johnson 1994). As public health scholar Amy Fairchild (2004) has described, immigrants arriving to the

United States in the early twentieth century were routinely inspected for diseases and were assessed for their overall health. Immigrants who were unhealthy, unfit for work, or exhibited signs of infectious disease, were not permitted entry into the United States (Fairchild 2004).

These historic anxieties about immigrants being a public charge have persisted, and public charge rhetoric has informed contemporary forms of blaming immigrants for US health system failures and shortcomings. For example, anti-immigrant rhetoric often hinges on claiming immigrants overuse and abuse public health and medical resources despite contrary evidence (Flavin et al. 2018). Public charge claims have also historically conflated health status, labor potential, and perceived racial differences. The same immigration policies that determined immigrants' ability to enter the United States were informed by assumptions about immigrants' racial and physical inferiority (Fairchild 2004). Indeed, race has prominently featured in immigration laws that have sought to ban certain types of immigrants from entering the United States (E. Lee 2002), and such efforts are not simply historic policy agendas; they became key features of immigration policy under the Trump administration.

While the United States historically denied immigrants' entry into the country based on race, health, perceived likelihood to become a public charge, and labor-readiness, the Trump administration doubled-down on long-standing logics of excluding immigrants from the United States. For example, the administration has passed a ban on immigrants from predominately Muslim countries from entering the country (colloquially known as the "Muslim ban"), and Trump repeatedly used racist rhetoric to build resentment against immigrants from Mexico and other Latin American countries, suggesting immigrants from those nations have a propensity for violent crime such as rape (M. Y. H. Lee 2015). In other words, the administration used the tropes of racial difference and perceived inferiority to guide its articulated stance on immigration. The conflated notions of race and perceived benefit to the country also guided the administration's proposals to redefine public charge policies.

In 2018, the Trump administration proposed altering existing public charge policies and broadening definitions for who could be considered a public charge. The proposed changes allowed for more easily denying immigrants' petitions for permanent legal resident status and immigration authorization based on family reunification (Henry J. Kaiser Family Foundation 2018). Prior to the Trump administration, immigrants were only considered to be a potential "public charge" if they used governmental cash assistance as a primary source of income (Parmet 2018). Under this application of the public charge policy, immigrants who received other benefits, such as publicly funded health insurance, were not considered a public charge (Parmet 2018). While undocumented immigrants are ineligible for publicly funded health services, documented immigrants are eligible for federally funded health services such as Medicaid, the nation's health program for low-income populations, after being lawfully present in the United States for five years (Henry J. Kaiser Family Foundation 2020). Moreover, authorized immigrants who meet the same five-year requirement are eligible to receive benefits through federal nutritional assistance programs such as Temporary Assistance for Needy Families (TANF) and Supplemental Nutrition Assistance Program (SNAP). TANF provides benefits for low-income families with children to cover basic expenses such as housing and childcare, and SNAP provides food assistance for low-income US residents.

Under changes that occurred during the Trump administration, non-citizens who receive benefits like SNAP or TANF in an amount greater than 15 percent of the federal poverty level could have been considered a public charge and potentially prohibited from adjusting their immigration status to become citizens or permanent residents (Enns and Ramirez 2018; Henry J. Kaiser Family Foundation 2018). Furthermore, the administration's changes considered use of housing assistance programs, receiving emergency medical services through Emergency Medicaid, and obtaining services through the federally funded children's health insurance program (CHIP), as potential causes for being considered a "public charge" (Parmet 2018). It also allowed immigration authorities to consider factors such as limited English language proficiency or conditions affecting immigrants' ability to work or attend school in their determinations about whether an immigrant would be a public charge (National Immigration Law Center 2018). These changes provided new forms of discretion for denying an immigrant's legal status adjustment and also demonstrated a public policy effort to constrain access to legal residency and citizenship for a subset of immigrants.

Although the Biden administration reversed the Trump-era public charge rules, the changes may have had sweeping health-related consequences for immigrants and citizens alike. Specifically, the policy could have had a "chilling effect" on the use of services among US-born children with immigrant parents or children in mixed-status families (Castañeda and Melo 2014; Viladrich 2012). An estimated 13 percent of US citizen children have a noncitizen immigrant parent (Henry J. Kaiser Family Foundation 2018), and the changes might have resulted in some parents not wanting to use health services for which their children are legally eligible due to fears of having that usage held against them when attempting to adjust their immigration status.

Even though the public charge changes corresponded to individuals and not household members (the public charge assessment is tied to the person who receives and uses the benefit, not others in the household), confusion about the changes may have resulted in household and family impacts. Indeed, some immigrant families chose not to enroll household members for Medicaid benefits due to fear of the immigration-related consequences (Henry J. Kaiser Family Foundation 2018; Parmet 2018). Avoiding services for which they are entitled may contribute to immigrants internalizing a sense of being undeserving of health services (see, for example, Willen 2012, 2014) because of their immigration status, indicating potentially hidden consequences of changing public charge definitions. In other words, following Willen and Cook's (this volume) explanation of how context informs deservingness debates, the public charge policy change may have provided additional legal context for creating an internalized sense of being undeserving to health services. More broadly, this legal content includes a growing effort to govern immigrants through fear, particularly through immigration law and enforcement practices (Kline 2017).

Fear and Militarization: US Immigration Enforcement Regimes

The proposed public charge changes fit into an aggressive and militarized immigration policy context in the United States. For example, the United States-Mexico border has become increasingly militarized in recent years through the use of drones, a growing number of armed agents, full-scale walls, and fencing (De León 2015). Furthermore, the militarized border has become a symbol for separating immigrants from non-immigrants, and Donald Trump used the border wall as a campaign tool to energize his supporters through the chant "build the wall" (Holpuch 2019; Plott 2019). In 2019, the Trump administration, and Trump personally, were so adamant about adding additional segments to the existing United States-Mexico border wall that the administration refused to pass a budget to keep the US government open, resulting in the US federal government closing for a record-breaking thirty-five days (Smith 2019).

More than a symbol and political rallying tool, however, the militarized United States-Mexico border is also a site of death and migrant suffering. As Jason De León (2015) has argued, the militarized United States-Mexico border intentionally funnels migrants from Mexico into the harshest and most remote conditions of the Sonoran Desert, increasing migrants' likelihood of death and disappearance. De León shows how the natural environment of the desert does the "dirty work" for the US federal government, as migrants become dehydrated, injured, or are attacked by wildlife or opportunistic criminals who prey on migrants' vulnerability. The militarized border and the deliberate use of the desert, then, have become a strategic "killing machine" for the state (2015: 3).

In addition to an increasingly militarized United States-Mexico border, the United States also features a patchwork of immigration laws that exist at a federal and state level and have health-related consequences. Although immigration enforcement powers are typically reserved for the federal government in the United States, several states have passed their own immigration enforcement laws that effectively make local police officers immigration enforcement agents (Kline 2019). These laws grant local police the authority to stop and arrest anyone suspected of being undocumented and have led to widespread claims of racial profiling (Kline 2017). Moreover, federal policies, such as Section 287(g) of the Immigration and Nationality Act, provide local police officers the authority to enforce federal immigration laws.

The 287(g) program started in 1996 as part of the Illegal Immigration Reform and Immigrant Responsibility Act (IIRIRA) and establishes memorandums of agreement between federal officials and local law enforcement officers to enforce immigration laws (Arnold 2007). In 2012, Immigration and Customs Enforcement (ICE)—the federal agency responsible for immigration matters—announced it would no longer renew agreements with local police since other enforcement tactics, such as Secure Communities, were effective and made 287(g) obsolete (US Immigration and Customs Enforcement 2012). Secure Communities is a fingerprint sharing program: every person taken into police custody has their fingerprints sent to a federal database to search for past crimes and their potential immigration status. If a fingerprint match is found, ICE has forty-eight hours to interview the detained person and determine their immigration status and potentially initiate the deportation process. All jurisdictions participate in the Secure Communities program, and to some degree, its goals are the same as the 287(g) program. In 2017, however, Donald Trump issued an executive order (Executive Order 13767: Border Security and Immigration Enforcement Improvements) to establish more 287(g) agreements, reversing the 2012 ICE decision. This reversal signaled an ongoing effort to use multiple and even redundant policies as a tool to threaten immigrants' stability in the United States and increase immigrants' concerns about deportation (Menjívar 2014). These, and other immigration enforcement laws, have a number of health-related consequences.

Immigration enforcement laws such as 287(g), and state-level policies that make local police de facto immigration agents increase immigrants' stress, fear, and anxiety, and result in avoiding health care when needed (Alexander and Fernandez 2014; Kline 2017; Rhodes et al. 2015; White et al. 2014). Moreover, specific immigration enforcement actions, such as raids, have been linked to adverse maternal and child health outcomes, including delivering low birthweight babies and being unable to lactate immediately following a raid (Lopez et al. 2017; Novak, Geronimus, and Martinez-Cardoso 2017). The combination of federal and state immigration statutes and local police practices has also had hidden consequences on health institutions on which all people rely. For example, in the US state of Georgia, immigration enforcement policies led some hospital employees to believe they had a "license to discriminate" against some immigrant patients, resulting in private hospitals sending those patients to public facilities without treatment, resulting in potentially higher health care costs overall and longer waiting times for all patients (Kline 2019).

In some US states, local municipalities have passed laws to create less hostile policy climates for immigrants to contradict state laws. These policies consist of more inclusive access to health care coverage, as demonstrated by the city of San Francisco allowing undocumented immigrants access to publicly funded services (Marrow 2012). Similarly, as Kristin Yarris (this volume) shows, state governments, including in Oregon, have actively combated federal immigration laws through creating "sanctuary policies." The federal government has challenged inclusive policies like those in San Francisco and Oregon, and other states have created their own efforts to preempt municipal sanctuary policies. For example, the state of Florida passed a law in 2019 that prohibits so-called sanctuary city policies or policies that municipal and local governments enact that broadly assert noncompliance with federal immigration agents (National Conference of State Legislatures 2019). This law, commonly referred to by its bill name Senate Bill (SB) 168, prohibits municipal governments from passing sanctuary city policies, creating legal tensions between the authority of local and state governments. Similar laws exist in eleven other states, and at the time of writing this chapter, twenty-one state legislatures were considering sanctuary city legislation (National Conference of State Legislatures 2019; Shoichet 2019). Conversely, nine US States have laws that do not infringe on sanctuary cities (National Conference of State Legislatures 2019), pointing to an inconsistent policy landscape that is contested in individual states and at a federal level.

The tensions surrounding enforcement and compliance with federal immigration agents have led some states to pursue legislation requiring individual law enforcement officers to cooperate with ICE officials. In North Carolina, for example, one proposed policy, House Bill (HB) 370, would require sheriffs across the state to work with ICE. As a result, sheriffs who were elected based on promises to cease 287(g) relationships are now feeling targeted by state legislators, and opponents of the law have specifically called it retaliation against officers who do not want to aggressively police immigrants in their communities (Carolina 2019; Burns 2019). Anti-sanctuary city policies and laws that force compliance with ICE, ultimately transform everyday residents into a system of state-level anti-immigrant surveillance. On a federal level, the Trump administration amplified this effort through Executive Order 13768: Enhancing Public Safety in the Interior of the United States, which threatens to terminate federal funding to locations that have any form of sanctuary policy (National Conference of State Legislatures 2019). Combined, these policies point to how the United States continues to promote an aggressive immigrant policing regime and attempts to govern immigrants through fear of detection and deportation.

Immigrant Detention: Profit, Family Separation, and Gender Violence

While the United States' immigration enforcement policies have deleterious health and social consequences on immigrants, their families, and their communities, these policies have proved profitable for a number of US corporations. Aggressive immigration enforcement laws have resulted in a burgeoning business for private prison corporations. Since 1999, the United States has continually privatized its incarceration system, and in doing so, grown the number of privatized immigration detention centers (Enns and Ramirez 2018). Private prisons and detention centers are a booming business: the two largest corporations, CoreCivic and Geo Group, operate 128 and 69 facilities respectively in the United States (Core Civic 2019a; The GEO Group 2018b), and immigration facilities account for the largest growth in the private prison industry (Enns and Ramirez 2018). In 2018, CoreCivic earned US$1.84 billion in revenue, and Geo Group earned US$2.3 billion (CoreCivic 2019b; The Geo Group 2018a). For detention centers, specifically, these profits occur in the context of detainee mistreatment. Inside the detention centers, detainees can be provided unhealthy and sometimes nutritionally insufficient food; are subject to harassment, physical and sexual abuse; and can be denied access to legal counsel, medical treatment, and even basic sanitary needs like clean clothing (Wright 2017). Being held in a detention center, then, can be harmful for immigrants' health but profitable for shareholders of private prison companies.

The health-related consequences of immigration detention in the United States gained notoriety under the Trump administration due to facility overcrowding and the strategic use of family separation. In 2017, Department of Homeland Security Director John Kelly announced a policy of separating children from parents as a way to deter immigrants crossing into the United States, fulfilling a Trump campaign promise to enact a policy that would "crackdown" on immigration (Davis and Shear

2019). The practice was part of the administration's overall "zero-tolerance" approach to immigration, which included border patrol agents vigilantly separating children who arrive with family members who are not their parents (Jordan and Dickerson 2019). When separated, children were held in overcrowded cells or cages and grouped by age or sex (Dickerson 2019). Notably, holding children in detention centers was not a new practice: during the Obama administration, unaccompanied minors who entered the United States were put into detention facilities and children who arrived with their parents were kept in family-specific facilities (Eagly, Shafer, and Whalley 2018; Schriro 2017). The Trump administration, however, augmented previous policies by deliberately separating parents from children and, during the process, failing to take appropriate measures to ensure family reunification (Soboroff 2019).

The conditions children were held in while detained were harmful to their health. Child detainees were denied basic hygienic needs such as soap, toothbrushes, shower facilities, and a change of clothing (Chapin 2019). Sleep hygiene was disrupted since the facilities were often overcrowded and child detainees were deprived of beds, thereby forcing them to sleep on the ground and often without blankets (Flynn 2019). Litigants who challenged these conditions claimed the US government violated the Flores agreement: a 1997 court settlement from a class action lawsuit about poor detention conditions, but the federal government defended the conditions in court, claiming hygienic items and clothing changes were not necessary (Montoya-Glavez 2019). Child detainees also reported physical and sexual abuse as well as harassment while in custody at detention facilities (Haag 2019). In some circumstances, children reported becoming temporary caretakers for other children—sometimes family members and sometimes strangers—who needed medical attention but did not receive it (Chapin 2019).

In addition to the unsanitary conditions of the facilities, parent-child separation due to immigration detention can also have lasting negative health consequences. Separation can cause long-term trauma, depression, and anxiety (Teicher 2018). Although federal authorities have claimed an attempt to reunite families, reports have surfaced that some children have been given to the wrong parents and some families are unable to be contacted (Bump 2018). For many immigrants, then, detention centers are a source of abuse, sickness, trauma, and long-term family separation. In some cases, they can even be sites of death. As of 2019, under the Trump administration, twenty-four migrants died while in the US government's custody (Rappleye and Seville 2019), and between September of 2018 and July of 2019 alone there were at least eleven deaths (Del Valle 2019).

The trauma and physical harms of detention centers are exacerbated by intersecting vulnerabilities such as being undocumented and identifying as lesbian, gay, bisexual, transgender, or otherwise queer-identifying (LGBTQ+). LGBTQ+ detainees may be especially exposed to mistreatment and harassment from staff and other detainees (Arriola and Raymond 2017), and intersecting forms of marginalization can potentially increase risk for medical maltreatment and death. For example, on 1 June 2019, Johana Medina Leon, a twenty-five-year-old transgender woman seeking asylum in the United States from El Salvador, died after being held for six weeks by ICE officials. Like thousands of other undocumented LGBTQ+ asylum seekers, Leon was held in a private, for profit, detention center notorious for poor treatment and unsafe conditions for LGBTQ+ migrants. She had tested positive for HIV and while in custody, ICE officials routinely denied her medical care (Levin 2019).

Leon's situation is not unusual, however; like Leon, other HIV-positive transgender women seeking asylum in the United States have died following release from ICE custody or while being detained (Fitzsimons 2918). LGBTQ+ Latinx migrants face precarious access to social services and are subjected to physical and sexual assault at disproportionately high rates compared to non-LGBTQ+ migrants (Hopkinson et al. 2017), and existing policies insufficiently protect them or respond to their needs. For example, transgender migrants are not necessarily able to be detained in facilities that match their gender identity, and there are no standard best-practice policies for how to protect LGBTQ+ detainees from abuse in detention centers. Moreover, as a result of the Trump administration's "remain in Mexico" policy, LGBTQ+ asylum seekers faced potentially disproportionate harm while seeking asylum in the United States.

The "remain in Mexico" policy, formally titled the Migrant Protection Protocols, allowed the US government to return asylum seekers to Mexico while they waited for a court hearing (United States Department of Homeland Security 2019). Prior to the Trump administration, asylum-seekers could wait for their hearings and stay in the United States, but the administration changed this process as part of an overall aggressive stance on denying immigrants entry into the country and an attempt to end what administration officials called "catching and releasing" migrants (Gonzales 2019). Between January of 2019, when the policy was enacted, and July of 2019, more than 12,000 migrants were sent to Mexico, and those asylum seekers were sometimes forced to stay in circumstances contributing to their insecurity (Sacchetti 2019). LGBTQ+ asylum seekers were particularly vulnerable since many of them encounter abuse, assault, and discrimination during their routes to the United States and while waiting for a court hearing (Kinosian and Partlow 2018).

Overall, immigrant detention practices, family separation policies, and the "remain in Mexico" policy result in deleterious health-related consequences for migrants and are specifically the result of efforts to "govern immigrants through crime," or as Jonathan Inda and Julie Dowling (2013: 2) explain, use crime and punishment as a way to control immigrants. Moreover, these policies construct ideas about who is considered a desirable immigrant, often based on perceived race and socioeconomic status. Defining desirability based on race and economic status magnified under the Trump administration, perhaps most notably under the announced end of the temporary protected status (TPS). TPS allows immigrants to remain in the United States when conditions in other countries are unsafe, such as suffering from civil conflict or natural disaster. The administration announced an end to TPS for immigrants from Haiti, El Salvador, Nicaragua, Sudan, Nepal, and Honduras, and a number of court challenges to the changes argued termination of TPS was based on racial discrimination.

Buying Residency/Citizenship

While the United States has made considerable efforts to exclude some immigrants, it has conversely made legal residency and citizenship easily accessible through financial investment. Immigration to the United States is not an easy process, and even immigrants who marry US citizens must wait years—sometimes apart from their spouses—before being granted residency (Gomberg-Muñoz 2016). However, there are immigration shortcuts available to wealthy individuals. Immigrants who invest US$500,000 in certain business can receive an EB-5 Visa, which grants them legal permanent residency and a fast track to citizenship, effectively allowing them to bypass hurdles and struggles other immigrants encounter by making large financial contributions to the US economy.

The EB-5 program is the United States' citizenship investment program—a way for the United States to attract wealthy global investors with the promise of US residency and citizenship. As Yossi Harpaz and Pablo Mateos argue, citizenship investment programs like the EB-5 create pathways for the wealthy to "circumvent restrictive immigration laws and policies" (2019: 848). The program started in 1990 and was intended to support rural areas or places with high unemployment rates (Lin 2014). The federal government caps the number of visas granted annually at 10,000, and in recent years, the EB-5 program has gotten national attention due to potential controversy surrounding the Trump administration. In 2017, the administration, and individual Trump family members, specifically, were criticized for flaunting the program to investors from China to demonstrate the ease of getting legal permanent residency in the United States (Rauhala and Wan 2017). Investigators examining Trump family members, including Donald Trump's son-in-law, Jared Kushner, have suggested Trump family members have used the office of the presidency and the EB-5 program as a way to entice investors into funding their own financial projects (Lipton and Drucker 2017). The Trump administration's alleged use of the program as a business tool underscores a chief concern with the program itself: that immigration matters have become commodified and could be used to support financial interests for a wealthy minority.

The United States is not the only country to offer authorized immigration status in exchange for significant financial investment. Several nations provide legal status or citizenship for investing large sums of money that can range from US$100,000 to several million dollars, and in the European Union (EU) alone twenty-three nation-states have immigration investment programs (Džankić 2018). These investments can provide significant financial boosts to some economies; in St. Kitt's, for example, passports provided through citizenship investments account for the large portions of the gross domestic product (van Fossen 2018). Depending on the nation, the programs can require establishing residence, such as in the United Kingdom, United States, Canada, Belgium, and Australia, or be more flexible with citizenship practices, as is the case in St. Kitts and Nevis and Dominica (Boatcă 2015). Overall, these types of investment programs can be grouped in two ways: programs that provide permanent residency and programs that provide full citizenship (Džankić 2018:

66). As Jelena Džankić argues, nation-states adopt these programs to attract enough investment that will improve their gross domestic product, seeking to either attract "long-distance residents" or "wealthy participants" in social and political life (2018: 74–75).

The residency programs and varying investor laws have partly given rise to citizenship investment corporations and concierge services in which clients interested in making citizenship investments hire someone like my airline seatmate to handle all aspects of the business transaction, including purchasing a place of residence. Some of the world's firms offering concierge services advertise benefits of "visa free travel" and rights and protections conferred to individuals by the state through citizenship by investment (CS Global Partners 2017). One of the leading citizenship-by-investment firms, Henley & Partners, reported a boom in both demand and supply of alternative citizenship programs (Henley & Partners 2019), reflecting a global trend in nations profiting from what their citizenship offers to wealthy individuals, and how wealthy investors can purchase rights and relationships with one or more nations.

Whereas citizenship as a legal relationship between the state and an individual was once characterized by exclusive allegiance to one nation-state, citizenship investment programs allow for dual, second, or additional citizenship that reflects global economic inequalities and alterations of identity (Harpaz and Mateos 2019). Collecting citizenship statuses can be a way for individuals to align themselves with a sense of place, identity, and family history, but citizenship investment programs, more specifically, serve strategic financial interests and can be a way to flaunt wealth. Among the global wealthy, such programs function to reduce tax burdens, and they have also become a trendy status symbol, as highlighted in online periodicals (Christians 2017; Millington 2018). Second citizenship, then, not only allows for a legal way to expedite immigration matters, but has also become a luxury accessory for a few, while any chance of legal authorization for non-wealthy immigrants can be limited.

Commodifying citizenship is not without governmental criticism, however. When Malta decided to sell passports and European citizenship for 650,000 euro in 2013, a debate in the European Parliament sparked about the right to become "European" based on income (Mavelli 2018). The debate about Malta revealed broader anxieties about how membership to one European country through investment ultimately granted access to all European countries that are EU members (Shachar and Baubock 2014).

The commodification of citizenship is an extension of historic ways of purchasing prestige, such as purchasing nobility and honors, and contributes to the contemporary formation of a global elite class (Tanasoca 2016). Further, the ability to buy legal residency and citizenship reflects a global economy of legal rights and protections that are available to only the wealthy. There is indeed a dichotomy of global privilege and freedom of movement associated with income, and this is also true in the United States. For example, the man I sat next to on the airplane noted that many of his clients were wealthy US residents concerned about the future of the country under Donald Trump's leadership. In particular, he noted some of his clients chose to find security through citizenship investment programs because they feared Trump reversing rights for LGBTQ+ populations: "A lot of my clients are wealthy gay guys who are freaked out about Trump and looking at their options to leave." Notably, the vulnerability of being LGBTQ+ may inform decisions to find alternative ideas of safety, but the fact that such alternatives are available to those who can afford them merits critique. Ironically, as the citizenship broker I sat next to on the plane suggested, the Trump administration's positions on social policies may have resulted in heightened fears among some populations, including wealthy LGBTQ+ individuals, effectively discouraging the very forms of financial investment that policies like the EB-5 attempt to promote. In other words, anxiety about Trump's social policies may have played a role in undermining the financialization efforts of the US immigration system by threatening investors' confidence in their own government's stability.

Financialization of Immigration System and Health System

Immigration investor programs point to how immigration processes in the United States and globally are becoming financialized. Social scientists use financialization as a theoretical frame to consider how social services have become infused with neoliberal market logics and become instruments for profit. Medical anthropologists, specifically, have used financialization theories to consider how health care systems and hospitals themselves have become financial instruments focused on generating revenue as part of the United States' market-based medical system (Kline 2018; Mulligan 2016). Through a growing financialization of immigration, and an existing financialization of health care, immigration and health in the United States are bound in a complex political and economic context.

In the United States, healthcare is largely treated as a commodity and not a right or social good. Most people obtain health services by obtaining insurance through their employer, but a large number of people are unable to obtain insurance and subsequent care. As the anthropologist Jessica Mulligan argues, the growing financialization of US health care systems can be observed through several factors, including (1) conversion of non-profit institutions into for-profit; (2) creating financial instruments to cover costs of care; (3) health care institutions; efforts to maximize revenue; (4) a focus on shareholder outcomes instead of health outcomes; and (5) a system of expansion, merger, and consolidation mirroring other forms of corporate profit-generating entities (2016: 39). Overall, the current US healthcare system results in deep inequalities in life expectancy and overall health status, and wealthy residents are more likely to live longer and report better health than low-income residents (Deaton 2002). Such inequalities speak to a core problem with financializing a necessary aspect of life: not everyone can afford the same basic level of care and potential treatment, resulting in deep health disparities in the United States (Braveman et al. 2010).

Just as the US healthcare system has become increasingly financialized, the citizenship investment opportunities described here demonstrate how immigration in the United States is similarly becoming financialized. This financial regime coexists alongside aggressive immigration regimes for those who are unable to invest large sums of money. Such a dichotomous system reflects deep socioeconomic and mobility inequalities, but also reflects broad efforts to alter the relationship between immigrants and the state.

The kinds of citizenship available to a global wealthy elite reflect a change in how overall sets of rights are not necessarily linked to the nation-state but instead to different types of political and economic factors (Aneesh and Wolover 2017). Social scientists examining the relationship between individuals and the state have used citizenship as a theoretical device to examine sets of rights and entitlements and how people make demands or assert rights (Isin and Turner 2002; Petryna 2002). The growing financialization of immigration that occurs in tandem with an already financialized US healthcare system suggests that immigrants must pay not only to participate in a health care system but also for their own security and freedom from aggressive immigration laws. The simultaneous financialization of immigration and ongoing financialization of health care in the United States thus signifies how basic rights such as a right to health and right to move continue to become commodities. The commodification of these rights ultimately restricts access to them for the wealthy. To summarize, just like the United States' financialized health care system that functions through a proverbial "pay to play" system, the financialized immigration system in the United States has created a "pay to stay" or "pay for flexibility to stay" regimen (Kim 2018).

Examined together, the financialization of health care and immigration policy reflects an overall effort to govern all immigrants through neoliberal aims (Mavelli 2018). As Luca Mavelli, borrowing from Michel Foucault, has argued, citizenship investment programs reformulate belonging in economic terms, transforming immigrants into "entrepreneurial actors," and by doing so, these policies advance the neoliberalization of all aspects of human life (2018: 483). Similarly, the financialization of US health care advances a neoliberal agenda for people in the United States to be self-reliant and secure their own health services (Maskovsky 2000; Rylko-Bauer and Farmer 2002). In effect, citizenship investment programs and the simultaneously operating harsh immigration regime that has also attempted to broaden definitions of public charge understandings, have served to create a "political economy of belonging" where immigration concerns are rewritten with a neoliberal logic (Mavelli 2018).

Needed Policy Interventions

The financialization of immigration and health care in the United States, along with the increasingly aggressive immigration enforcement regimes, demand policy changes. At the federal level, both immigration and health reform are necessary to combat neoliberal models of financing health services and immigration laws that conflate race, health, and income. Federal immigration law changes include a needed comprehensive immigration reform that provides pathways to citizenship for undocumented immigrants currently in the United States and alter the current citizenship and legal residency regime that benefits wealthy investors. Furthermore, as several anthropologists have argued, the aggressive immigration enforcement regime that harms immigrants' health and has extended health-related consequences on immigrants' family members must end. This includes ceasing family separation and militarized border enforcement tactics and the forms of routine enforcement that occur through policies such as 287(g).

Additionally, addressing the financialization of immigration laws and militarization of enforcement requires policies that respond to private prisons and detention centers. The types of abuses that occur in private prisons and detention centers are an amalgam of profit-driven motivation and lack of oversight, and such efforts demand immediate intervention. Similarly, preemption laws that that prohibit creating inclusive policies for immigrants must continue to be challenged in US courts, and individual voters must hold their legislators accountable for proposing or passing such laws. Accordingly, litigation and political mobilization as a way to advance policy change may prove an effective strategy to reverse harsh immigration regimes, and anthropologists are positioned to aid in such efforts by explaining the lived consequences of immigration legislation.

While the scenarios identified here demand long-term solutions, there are more immediate solutions possible. For example, current immigrant rights organizations can pressure detention centers and ICE to be attentive to the unique needs of LGBTQ+ migrants and keep them safe from harassment and abuse. Moreover, these organizations could call for changing EB-5 programs and broadening immigration policies to be inclusive of immigrants who do not make significant financial investments. These efforts would help contribute to policy reforms that move beyond the financial logics that partly undergird immigration and health policy.

Conclusion

As divisive immigration politics continue on a global scale and are reflected through political efforts like Brexit and persistent attention to the United States-Mexico border wall, anthropologists must play a role in challenging anti-immigrant policies. Anthropologists who make law and policy an ethnographic field to be studied can document how policy creates unique inequalities and lived experiences (Wedel et al. 2005), and can use policy as a means for changing systems of inequality. In this respect, documenting and challenging policy as a cause of inequality and poor health, in particular, can advance efforts to correct systemic injustices.

Nolan Kline is an assistant professor in the Department of Health Behavior and Health Systems at the University of North Texas Health Science Center. His book, *Pathogenic Policing: Immigration Enforcement and Health in the US South* (Rutgers), describes the multiple health-related consequences of immigration enforcement policies and police practices in Atlanta, Georgia. His current research focuses on LGBTQ+ Latinx activism following the Pulse shooting in Orlando, Florida, and is supported by the National Science Foundation. As an applied medical anthropologist, his work overlaps with public health, law, and policy.

References

Alexander, William L., and Magdalena Fernandez. 2014. "Immigration Policing and Medical Care for Farmworkers: Uncertainties and Anxieties in the East Coast Migrant Stream." *North American Dialogue* 17(1): 13–30.

Aneesh, A., and David J. Wolover. 2017. "Citizenship and Inequality in a Global Age." *Sociology Compass* 11(5): e12477.

Arnold, Carrie L. 2007. "Racial Profiling in Immigration Enforcement: State and Local Agreements to Enforce Federal Immigration Law." *Ariz. l. rev.* 49: 113–42.

Arriola, Elvia R., and Virginia M. Raymond. 2017. "Migrants Resist Systemic Discrimination and Dehumanization in Private, For-Profit Detention Centers." *Santa Clara J. Int'l L.* 15: 1–42.

Boatcă, Manuela. 2015. "Commodification of Citizenship: Global Inequalities and the Modern Transmission of Property. " In *Overcoming Global Inequalities*, ed. Immanuel Wallerstein and Christopher Chase-Dunn, 13–28. London: Routledge.

Braveman, Paula A., Catherine Cubbin, Susan Egerter, David R. Williams, and Elsie Pamuk. 2010. "Socioeconomic Disparities in Health in the United States: What the Patterns Tell Us." *American Journal of Public Health* 100(S1): S186–S196.

Bump, Philip. 2018. "The Children Separated from their Parents, by the Numbers." Retrieved 2 January 2019 from https://www.washingtonpost.com/news/politics/wp/2018/07/09/the-children-separated-from-their-parents-by-the-numbers/?utm_term=.8d5b705fdb40.

Burns, Matthew. 2019. "Metro Sheriffs Feel Targeted by Legislation Requiring Ice Relationship." *WRAL News*. June 19. https://www.wral.com/metro-sheriffs-feel-targeted-by-legislation-requiring-ice-relationship/18461017/

Carolina, A. C. L. U. o. N. 2019. "Hb 370—Require Sheriff Cooperation with ICE." Retrieved 25 July 2019 from https://www.acluofnorthcarolina.org/en/legislation/hb-370-require-sheriff-cooperation-ice.

Castañeda, Heide, and Milena Andrea Melo. 2014. "Health Care Access for Latino Mixed-Status Families. Barriers, Strategies, and Implications for Reform." *American Behavioral Scientist* 58(14): 1891–1909.

Chapin, Angela. 2019. "In Their Own Words, Migrant Children Describe Horrific Conditions at Border Patrol Facilities." Retrieved 21 June 2021 from https://www.huffpost.com/entry/migrant-children-describe-detention_n_5d1646ffe4b03d61163af666.

Christians, Allison. 2017. "Buying In: Residence and Citizenship by Investment." *St Louis ULJ* 62: 51–72.

Core Civic. 2019a. "Find a Facility." Retrieved 23 July 2019 from http://www.corecivic.com/facilities.

———. 2019b. "Corecivic Reports Fourth Quarter and Full Year 2018 Financial Results." Retrieved 23 July 2019 from http://ir.corecivic.com/node/20366/pdf.

CS Global Partners. 2017. "Citizenship Solutions and Investment Programmes." Retrieved 26 July 2019 from https://csglobalpartners.com/citizenship-solutions/.

Davis, Julie H., and Michael D. Shear. 2019. "How Trump Came to Enforce a Practice of Separating Migrant Families." *The New York Times*, 16 June 2018. Retrieved 21 June 2021 from https://www.nytimes.com/2018/06/16/us/politics/family-separation-trump.html.

De León, Jason. 2015. *The Land of Open Graves: Living and Dying on the Migrant Trail.* Berkeley: University of California Press.
Deaton, Angus. 2002. "Policy Implications of the Gradient of Health and Wealth." *Health Affairs* 21(2): 13–30.
Del Valle, Gaby. 2019. "A Honduran Man Just Died in Immigration Custody. He's the 11th since September." *Vice News*, 2 July 2019.
Dickerson, Caitlin. 2019. "'There Is a Stench': Soiled Clothes and No Baths for Migrant Children at a Texas Center." *The New York Times*, 21 June 2019. Retrieved 21 June 2021 from https://www.nytimes.com/2019/06/21/us/migrant-children-border-soap.html.
Džankić, Jelena. 2018. "Immigrant Investor Programmes in the European Union (EU)." *Journal of Contemporary European Studies* 26(1): 64–80.
Eagly, Ingrid, Steven Shafer, and Jana Whalley. 2018. "Detaining Families: A Study of Asylum Adjudication in Family Detention." *Calif. L. Rev.* 106: 785–868.
Enns, Peter K., and Mark D. Ramirez. 2018. "Privatizing Punishment: Testing Theories of Public Support for Private Prison and Immigration Detention Facilities." *Criminology* 56(3): 546–73.
Fairchild, Amy L. 2004. "Policies of Inclusion: Immigrants, Disease, Dependency, and American Immigration Policy at the Dawn and Dusk of the 20th Century." *American Journal of Public Health* 94(4): 528–39.
Fitzsimons, Tim. 2018. "Transgender Ice Detainee Died of Aids Complications, Autopsy Shows." *NBC News*, 17 April 2019. Retrieved 21 June 2021 from https://www.nbcnews.com/feature/nbc-out/transgender-ice-detainee-died-aids-complications-autopsy-shows-n994836.
Flavin, Lila, Leah Zallman, Danny McCormick, and J. Wesley Boyd. 2018. "Medical Expenditures on and by Immigrant Populations in the United States: A Systematic Review." *International Journal of Health Services* 48(4): 601–21.
Flynn, M. 2019. "Detained Migrant Children Got No Toothbrush, No Soap, No Sleep. No Problem, Government Argues." *Washington Post.* June 21. https://www.texastribune.org/2019/06/21/detained-migrant-children-no-toothbrush-no-soap/
Gomberg-Muñoz, Ruth. 2016. *Becoming Legal: Immigration Law and Mixed Status Families.* Oxford: Oxford University Press.
Gonzales, Richard. 2019. "U.S. Is Rolling Out Its 'Remain in Mexico' Policy on Central American Asylum-Seekers." *National Public Radio*, 24 January 2019. Retrieved 21 June 2021 from https://www.npr.org/2019/01/24/688470513/u-s-plans-to-enforce-remain-in-mexico-policy-on-central-american-asylum-seekers?t=1624308543480.
Haag, Matthew. 2019. "Thousands of Immigrant Children Said They Were Sexually Abused in U.S. Detention Centers, Report Says." *The New York Times*, 27 February 2019. Retrieved 21 June 2021 from https://www.nytimes.com/2019/02/27/us/immigrant-children-sexual-abuse.html.
Harpaz, Yossi, and Pablo Mateos. 2019. "Strategic Citizenship: Negotiating Membership in the Age of Dual Nationality." *Journal of Ethnic and Migration Studies* 45(6): 843–57.
Henley & Partners. 2019. "A Guide to Investment Migration for Governments and Global Citizens." Retrieved 26 July 2019 from https://www.henleyglobal.com/files/download/guide-to-investment-migration-for-overnments-and-global-citizens-01–2019.pdf.
Henry J. Kaiser Family Foundation. 2018. "Proposed Changes to 'Public Charge' Policies for Immigrants: Implications for Health Coverage." Retrieved 21 June 2021 from https://files.kff.org/attachment/Issue-Brief-Proposed-Changes-to-Public-Charge-Policies-for-Immigrants-Implications-for-Health-Coverage.
———. 2020. "Health Coverage of Immigrants: Disparities Policy." Retrieved 21 June 2021

from https://www.kff.org/racial-equity-and-health-policy/fact-sheet/health-coverage-of-immigrants/.

Holpuch, Amanda. 2019. "What Exactly Is Trump's Border Wall and Why Does He Want $5.7bn for It?" *The Guardian*, 15 January 2019. Retrieved 21 June 2021 from https://www.theguardian.com/us-news/2019/jan/15/trump-mexico-border-wall-status-migrants.

Hopkinson, Rebecca A., Eva Keatley, Elizabeth Glaeser, Laura Erickson-Schroth, Omar Fattal, and Melba Nicholson Sullivan. 2017. "Persecution Experiences and Mental Health of LGBT Asylum Seekers." *Journal of Homosexuality* 64(12): 1650–66.

Inda, Jonathan Xavier, and Julie A. Dowling. 2013. "Introduction: Governing Migrant Illegality." In *Governing Immigration through Crime*, ed. Jonathan Xavier Inda and Julie A. Dowling. Stanford, CA: Stanford University Press.

Isin, Engin F., and Bryan S. Turner. 2002. "Citizenship Studies: An Introduction." In *Handbook of Citizenship Studies*, ed. Ensin F. Isin and B. S. Turner. London: Sage Publications Ltd.

Johnson, Kevin R. 1994. "Public Benefits and Immigration: The Intersection of Immigration Status, Ethnicity, Gender, and Class." *UCLA L. Rev.* 42: 1–35.

Jordan, M., and C. Dickerson. 2019. "Hundreds of Migrant Children Are Taken from Families Despite Rollback of Separation Policy." *The Boston Globe*. March 9. https://www.bostonglobe.com/news/nation/2019/03/09/hundreds-migrant-children-are-taken-from-families-despite-rollback-separation-policy/qRgH3JRc8G7KEgzQz5aHfO/story.html?__twitter_impression=true&outputType=amp

Kim, Jaeeun. 2018. "Migration-Facilitating Capital: A Bourdieusian Theory of International Migration." *Sociological Theory* 36(3): 262–88.

Kinosian, Sarah, and Joshua Partlow. 2018. "LGBT Asylum Seekers First to Reach U.S. Border from Caravan. Now They Wait." *The Washington Post*. November 13. https://www.washingtonpost.com/world/the_americas/the-first-caravan-migrants-arrive-at-the-us-border-and-begin-the-waiting-game/2018/11/13/ceef3844-e6b7-11e8-8449-1ff263609a31_story.html.

Kline, Nolan. 2017. "Pathogenic Policy: Immigrant Policing, Fear, and Parallel Medical Systems in the US South." *Medical Anthropology* 36(4): 396–410.

______. 2018. "Life, Death, and Dialysis: Medical Repatriation and Liminal Life among Undocumented Kidney Failure Patients in the United States." *PoLAR: Political and Legal Anthropology Review* 41(2): 216–30.

______. 2019. *Pathogenic Policing: Immigration Enforcement and Health in the US South*. New Brunswick, NJ: Rutgers University Press.

Lee, Erika. 2002. "The Chinese Exclusion Example: Race, Immigration, and American Gatekeeping, 1882–1924." *Journal of American Ethnic History* 3: 36–62.

Lee, M. Y. H. 2015. "Donald Trump's False Comments Connecting Mexican Immigrants and Crime." *The Washington Post*. July 8. https://www.washingtonpost.com/news/fact-checker/wp/2015/07/08/donald-trumps-false-comments-connecting-mexican-immigrants-and-crime/

Levin, Sam. 2019. "Trans Woman Who Died after Illness in US Custody Had Asked to Be Deported, Family Says." *The Guardian*, 3 June 2019. Retrieved 21 June 2021 from https://www.theguardian.com/us-news/2019/jun/03/trans-migrant-dies-ice-us-immigration-johana-leon.

Lin, Annie Anjung. 2014. "Splitting the EB-5 Program: A Proposal for Employment-Based Immigration Reform to Better Target Immigrant Entrepreneurs and Investors." *Chap. L. Rev.* 18: 527–52.

Lipton, Eric, and Jesse Drucker. 2017. "Kushner Family Stands to Gain from Visa Rules in Trump's First Major Law." *The New York Times*, 8 May 2017.
Lopez, William D., Daniel J. Kruger, Jorge Delva, Mikel Llanes, Charo Ledón, Adreanne Waller, Melanie Harner, Ramiro Martinez, Laura Sanders, Margaret Harner, and Barbara Israel. 2017. "Health Implications of an Immigration Raid: Findings from a Latino Community in the Midwestern United States." *Journal of Immigrant and Minority Health* 19(3): 702–8.
Marrow, Helen B. 2012. "Deserving to a Point: Unauthorized Immigrants in San Francisco's Universal Access Healthcare Model." *Social Science & Medicine* 74(6): 846–54.
Maskovsky, Jeff. 2000. "Managing the Poor: Neoliberalism, Medicaid HMOs and the Triumph of Consumerism Among the Poor." *Medical Anthropology* 19(2): 121–46.
Mavelli, Luca. 2018. "Citizenship for Sale and the Neoliberal Political Economy of Belonging." *International Studies Quarterly* 62(3): 482–93.
Menjívar, Cecilia. 2014. "The 'Poli-Migra' Multilayered Legislation, Enforcement Practices, and Can We Learn about and from Today's Approaches." *American Behavioral Scientist* 58(13): 1–15.
Millington, Alison. 2018. "23 Countries Where Money Can Buy You a Second Passport or 'Elite Residency.'" *Business Insider*, 8 September 2018.
Montoya-Glavez, Camilo. 2019. "Here's Why the Trump Administration Says It's Not Required to Give Migrant Children Soap." *CBS News*, 24 June 2019.
Mulligan, Jessica. 2016. "Insurance Accounts: The Cultural Logics of Health Care Financing." *Medical Anthropology Quarterly* 30(1): 37–61.
National Conference of State Legislatures. 2019. "What's a Sanctuary Policy? FAQ on Federal, State and Local Action on Immigration Enforcement." Retrieved 23 July 2019 from http://www.ncsl.org/research/immigration/sanctuary-policy-faq635991795.aspx.
National Immigration Law Center. 2018. "Proposed Changes to the Public Charge Rule." Retrieved 23 July 2019 from https://www.nilc.org/issues/economic-support/pubcharge/proposed-changes-to-public-charge-rule-faq/.
Novak, Nicole L., Arline T. Geronimus, and Aresha M. Martinez-Cardoso. 2017. "Change in Birth Outcomes among Infants Born to Latina Mothers after a Major Immigration Raid." *International Journal of Epidemiology* 46(3): 839–49.
Parmet, Wendy. 2018. "The Health Impact of the Proposed Public Charge Rules." *Health Affairs Blog September* 27: 2018.
Petryna, Adriana. 2002. *Life Exposed: Biological Citizens after Chernobyl.* Princeton, NJ: Princeton University Press.
Plott, Elaina. 2019. "Trump Supporters Don't Make Chants about Men." *The Atlantic*, 19 July 2019.
Rappleye, Hannah, and Lisa Riordan Seville. 2019. "24 Immigrants Have Died in Ice Custody during the Trump Administration." *NBC News*, 9 June 2019. Retreived 21 June 2021 from https://www.nbcnews.com/politics/immigration/24-immigrants-have-died-ice-custody-during-trump-administration-n1015291.
Rauhala, Emilie, and W. Wan. 2017. "In a Beijing Ballroom, Kushner Family Pushes $500,000 'Investor Visa' to Wealthy Chinese." *The Washington Post*, 6 May 2017.
Rhodes, Scott D., Lilli Mann, F. M. Simán, Eunyoung Song, Jorge Alonzo, Mario Downs, Emma Lawlor, Omar Martinez, Christina J. Sun, Marie Claire O'Brien, Beth A. Reboussin, and Mark A. Hall. 2015. "The Impact of Local Immigration Enforcement Policies on the Health of Immigrant Hispanics/Latinos in the United States." *American Journal of Public Health* 105(2): 329–37.

Rylko-Bauer, Barbara, and Paul Farmer. 2002. "Managed Care or Managed Inequality? A Call for Critiques of Market-Based Medicine." *Medical Anthropology Quarterly* 16(4): 476–502.

Sacchetti, Maria. 2019. "U.S. Asylum Officers Urge Court to End Trump's 'Remain in Mexico' Policy." *The Washington Post*, 27 June 2019.

Schriro, Dora. 2017. "Weeping in the Playtime of Others: The Obama Administration's Failed Reform of Ice Family Detention Practices." *Journal on Migration and Human Security* 5(2): 452–80.

Shachar, A., and R. Baubock. 2014. "Should Citizenship Be For Sale?" Robert Schuman Centre for Advanced Studies Research Paper (2014/01).

Shoichet, Catherine E. 2019. "Florida Just Banned Sanctuary Cities. At Least 11 Other States Have, Too." *CNN Politics*, 14 June 2019.

Smith, David. 2019 "Trump Inches Closer to Declaring Emergency for Wall as Negotiations Stall." *The Guardian*, 31 January 2019.

Soboroff, Jacob. 2019. "Emails Show Trump Admin Had 'No Way to Link' Separated Migrant Children to Parents." *NBC News*. March 1. https://www.nbcnews.com/politics/immigration/emails-show-trump-admin-had-no-way-link-separated-migrant-n1000746.

Tanasoca, Ana. 2016. "Citizenship for Sale: Neomedieval, Not Just Neoliberal?" *European Journal of Sociology/Archives européennes de sociologie* 57(1): 169–95.

Teicher, Martin H. 2018. "Childhood Trauma and the Enduring Consequences of Forcibly Separating Children from Parents at the United States Border." *BMC Medicine* 16(1): 146.

The Geo Group. 2018a. "Annual Report." Retrieved 23 July 2019 from http://www.snl.com/interactive/newlookandfeel/4144107/GEOGroup2018AR.pdf.

———. 2018b. "Our Locations." Retrieved 23 July 2019 from https://www.geogroup.com/LOCATIONS.

US Immigration and Customs Enforcement. 2012. "Fy 2012: Ice Announces Year-End Removal Numbers, Highlights Focus on Key Priorities and Issues New National Detainer Guidance to Further Focus Resources." Retrieved 23 July 2019 from https://www.ice.gov/news/releases/fy-2012-ice-announces-year-end-removal-numbers-highlights-focus-key-priorities-and#wcm-survey-target-id.

United States Department of Homeland Security. 2019. "Migrant Protection Protocols." Retrieved 21 June 2021 from https://www.dhs.gov/news/2019/01/24/migrant-protection-protocols.

van Fossen, Anthony. 2018. "Passport Sales: How Island Microstates Use Strategic Management to Organise the New Economic Citizenship Industry." *Island Studies Journal* 13(1): 285–300.

Viladrich, Anahí. 2012. "Beyond Welfare Reform: Reframing Undocumented Immigrants' Entitlement to Health Care in the United States, a Critical Review." *Social Science & Medicine* 74(6): 822–29.

Wedel, Janine R., Cris Shore, Gregory Feldman, and Stacy Lathrop. 2005. "Toward an Anthropology of Public Policy." *The Annals of the American Academy of Political and Social Science* 600(1): 30–51.

White, Kari, Valérie A. Yeager, Nir Menachemi, and Isabel C. Scarinci. 2014. "Impact of Alabama's Immigration Law on Access to Health Care among Latina Immigrants and Children: Implications for National Reform." *American Journal of Public Health* 104(3): 397–405.

Willen, Sarah S. 2012. "How Is Health-Related 'Deservingness' Reckoned? Perspectives from Unauthorized Im/migrants in Tel Aviv." *Social Science & Medicine* 74(6): 812–21.

———. 2014. "Lightning Rods in the Local Moral Economy: Debating Unauthorized Migrants' Deservingness in Israel." *International Migration* 53(3): 70–86.
Wright, Jessica. 2017. "The Cost of (Non) Compliance: An Expose of the United States' Immigration Detention Policy and Its Failure to Comply with International Standards on Torture." *Intercultural Hum. Rts. L. Rev.* 12: 315–38.

8
Narrative Testimony and Political Potentiality
Surviving Family Separation, Advocating for Migrants' Rights and Well-being

Kristin Elizabeth Yarris

Public Testimony and Local Advocacy in Hostile Times

One late afternoon in February 2019, deep into Oregon's dark, wet winter, hundreds of community members filed into a downtown municipal government building, shaking rain off their hooded jackets as they entered. Inside the building doors, a line was forming as people waited to enter the large public hearing room that sat at the front of the building behind double doors. Two county workers sat at a folding table asking community members as they filed into the hearing whether they would like to sign up to give public testimony. As community members unzipped their rain jackets, T-shirts were revealed, emblazoned with slogans such as "Families Belong Together" and "#Ní Una Más" in reference to the nationwide movements in solidarity with immigrant communities and against family separations and deportations that were occurring across the United States since the prior year. The hearing of the County Board of Supervisors had been called with one main agenda item—allowing the public to register their views related to the County Sherriff's recent collaboration with federal immigration enforcement activities. Local news outlets had reported that the sheriff was allowing Immigration and Customs Enforcement (ICE) officers access to the county jail, permitting ICE to detain people newly released from the sheriff's custody. The immigrant rights groups that called for public participation in the hearing argued that the sheriff's practice violated Oregon's statewide "sanctuary" law, which has been on the books since 1987, as well as county and city sanctuary ordinances that were passed in 2018. Many community members packing into the public hearing were showing solidarity with communities vulnerable to deportation and family separation, others were directly impacted by heightened immigration enforcement. As an anthropologist concerned with transnational migration and health and as a public health professional engaged with local migrant solidarity work in Oregon, I participated in the public hearing both as a concerned community member and as a scholar interested in the ways local political organizing efforts were responding to federal policies hostile to migrants in ways that used sanctuary policies as a background through which to foster welcome and well-being for (im)migrant communities.

In this chapter, I draw on this public hearing as a site of engaged ethnography and an opportunity for an analysis of the ways activists are utilizing state and local policies related to sanctuary as a means of fostering new forms of political subjectivity and community belonging. As I show below, local community organizing efforts on behalf of migrant rights in the United States are able to draw on state and local sanctuary policies as a framework within which to cast their broader articulations of rights to membership, belonging, inclusion, and well-being. In particular, in the narrative testimony I analyze here, activists transform the space of the public hearing as a space of political possibility, situating themselves on the front lines of struggles for migrant justice and inclusion. In this space, public testimony becomes a narrative modality through which activists and community members reposition themselves, moving from narratives of "victims of family separation"—or from subject positions vulnerable to deportation and state violence of forced family separation—to a resignified political subjectivity that powerfully asserts a right to belong as visible members of the political community.

Viewing health and mental health as nested within multiple levels of influence is key to understanding health and well-being concerns among migrant communities. As the introduction to this volume asserts, public policies and social attitudes toward migrants, especially during hostile political eras, are two key influences on the health and well-being of individuals and families. Here, I focus on family separation policies as one dimension of a broader social and political climate of exclusion and hostility to immigrants. These exclusionary policies enact state violence on individual bodies, restricting mobility and enforcing removal (Kline 2019). In turn, the impact of social policies toward migrants have reverberating effects through families and communities (Lopez 2019).

The ethnographic focus of this chapter is the testimony given by community activists in protest of local law enforcement's collaboration with ICE. In particular, as a participant-observer and engaged anthropologist at the hearing, I was struck by a powerful narrative (re)framing that was reiterated by speakers in their public testimony, as community members and activists drew on their embodied positionality as "victims of family separation" to articulate claims to political belonging, membership, and well-being. In what follows then, I situate this narrative framing both within a brief review of anthropological work on testimony, and within the broader political context surrounding the 2019 public hearing—both US federal policies related to family separation and immigration enforcement and state and local policies in Oregon that seek to protect migrant families and communities.

Narrative Testimony: Resignifying Victimhood

Recent scholarship in migration and refugee studies has pivoted from solely focusing on suffering and victimhood toward emphasizing migrants' hopes, aspirations, and desires (see Carling and Collins 2018; Kvittingen et al. 2018; Watters 2019). This analytical move, while conceptually productive, is not without a political cost, as political and legal recognition of migrants and refugees within nation-state political and legal regimes is often predicated upon grounds of suffering and victimhood. For instance, in the United States, determination of asylum claims is based on "credible fear interviews," through which administrative officers of the state (usually, Customs and Border Patrol agents) capriciously allocate political rights to asylum based on determinations of persecution and violence in home countries (US Citizenship and Immigration Services 2015; Musalo 2019). In this framing, social protection and political rights for migrants are rendered by states along lines of suffering, with greater perceived hardships made the arbiter for rights and protection (Yarris and Castañeda 2015). Furthermore, as Didier Fassin and Estelle d'Halluin (2005) have argued, where states allocate rights on the basis of suffering, migrants' bodies themselves become the grounds upon which victimhood becomes visible, with claims to political membership often legitimated by medical authorities whose expertise strips agency from migrants themselves.

Within this political framing of migrant deservingness, narrative testimony plays a particular role in making suffering visible. Within the framework of immigration law, narrative testimonies often serve a particular function: registering the suffering of individual migrants/refugees/asylum seekers in order to lay claim to rights and protections from host states. Along these lines, Erica Caple James (2004) described how Haitian victims of political violence are encouraged to present a particular narrative of suffering and trauma to be deemed both eligible for assistance within the international humanitarian regime and recognized as political subjects. Examining the narratives produced through asylum hearings for African migrants in Belgium, Jan Bloommaert (2001) documents how the hearing's narrative structure situated migrants as victims in need of state protection, privileging a particular mode of truth-telling that focused on violence and victimhood while simultaneously fostering suspicion about the veracity of migrants' stories of displacement.

Thus, migrant testimony may act to reinforce social and political inequalities between migrants and host states, especially when it acts to strip speakers of agency and grants citizenship rights on the basis of suffering and victimhood. This "narrative inequality" (Bloommaert 2001: 415) is reaffirmed by the enforced dichotomy between economic migrants—viewed as willfully moving in search of better opportunities—and refugees, who are viewed as forced to move due to insecurity and violence (Yarris and Castañeda 2015). These legal and political dichotomies elide the very complicated realities of migratory movements, which transcend a simple division between elective and forced migration. And yet, this dichotomy between deserving and undeserving migrants is reinforced by the asylum process in the United States, where legal processes predicated on determinations of suffering require asylum seekers to repeatedly narrate their stories of hardship in order to be deemed credible as subjects deserving of rights and protection.

While narrative testimony can reinforce political categories, such testimony also harbors political potential to invert inscriptions of victimhood. For instance, Charles Briggs has eloquently analyzed the possibilities of testimony to generate new social possibilities beyond victimhood (Briggs 1997, 2007). Briggs focuses on the testimony of an indigenous Warao woman, Ms. Gómez, who is asked to testify in response to charges of infanticide leveled against her. Briggs shows how Ms. Gómez's testimony inverts expected narrative forms and resituates her subject position as an agent and survivor of social and political violence, rather than a powerless victim or a perpetrator of violence herself. Briggs states "Ms. Gómez's story became a story about . . . her own constraints as a narrator, and the profound consequence of [other people's] stories" in her own story (Briggs 2007: 316). Through his critical and self-reflective analysis, Briggs shows the power of testimony to unsettle the "natural grounding" of victimhood, as Ms. Gómez's account "opened up new insights into the very grounds by which violence can be narrativized" (Briggs 2007: 317).

Narrative testimony also has the potential of reframing historical events to move beyond individual impacts and shape collective perspectives and experiences. For instance, Lynn Stephen (2017) has reflected on the ways narrative testimony broadens anthropological analysis and influences public perceptions of historical events. Drawing from her long career of engaged research in various Latin American settings, as well as her advocacy in providing expert witness on asylum claims in US immigration courts, Stephen argues that oral testimony can become a mode of decolonizing knowledge production, as speakers demand rights to be heard by broader publics and these publics in turn assume the position of listeners.

This chapter is inspired by the political potential of narrative testimony to alter anticipated narrative framings of migrants-as-victims. In particular, in what follows, I show how public testimony can be a space through which migrants challenge their "assigned subject positions" (Briggs 2007: 316) as mere victims and assert their rights as political subjects. In the testimony analyzed here, which traces the impacts of state policies that have forcibly separated migrant families, the intersubjective and intergenerational aspect of narrative testimony becomes apparent. The speakers I document herein call out the impact of family separation policies not just for themselves, but for their extended families and communities. These narrative testimonies, performed in a public hearing where the audience includes elected municipal representatives, also have the potential of inverting power dynamics between citizens and non-citizens, insofar as migrants assert their right to belong. In other words, the political potential of narrative testimony is also on display, as migrants use testimony not only to reinforce their positionality as victims of state policy and state violence, but to assert their agency as political actors and their rights as political subjects.

State Violence, Family Separation, and Migrant Well-Being

The forced separation of families has a long and unfortunate history in the United States, but it has re-emerged in the current era as an explicit strategy of deterrence within an anti-immigrant federal policy regime. Since 2017, the US Department of Homeland Security has implemented a practice of separating families (children from parents or guardians) crossing into the country at the southern border. As part of the Department of Justice's "Zero Tolerance Policy" for unauthorized immigration, this "family separation policy" became official practice, resulting in thousands of children separated from their parents and detained in deplorable conditions in privately run immigrant detention centers (US Department of Justice 2018; US Department of Health and Human Services 2019). As journalists and media outlets exposed the impacts of the family separation policy, often through vivid images of detained and distressed children, responses ensued—in the form of popular outcry, civil litigation, and public protests across the country (Yoon-Hendricks and Greenberg 2018). I attended one such protest in the summer of 2018 in the city where I live in Oregon, where local immigrants' rights groups rallied alongside environmentalists, healthcare providers, Native American groups, and self-described "mothers with children" in an ad hoc coalition brought together under the banner of "Families Belong Together" (Families Belong Together 2019). The hundreds of community members, activists, and allies who showed up on short notice in downtown Eugene in protest of a federal immigration policy was evidence of the ways in which "family separation" had reentered the public consciousness as a discursive embodiment of state violence against migrant families and communities.

Researchers from various disciplines have documented the negative consequences of family separation on the health and well-being of children and youth in particular (for example, see Zayas et al. 2015). Such consequences include uncertainty, fear, anxiety, trauma, stress, and even suicidality (Zayas 2015; Habbach, Hampton, and Mishori 2020). In my prior work with Nicaraguan transnational families, I observed both children's astute awareness and understanding of the reasons for their parents' migrations, as well as an embodiment of the uncertainty and ambivalence surrounding potential reunification with parents abroad (Yarris 2014). Of course, the emotional distress of transnational family life is aggravated by policies that reinforce prolonged separation and complicate legal reunification. In the Nicaraguan families I work with, I have shown how this distress appears in embodied forms as the pain of "thinking too much" ("pensando mucho"), shared across generations by children, migrant mothers, and grandmother caregivers (Yarris 2017). While acknowledging the real consequences of family separation for children's well-being, I have also been careful not to pathologize transnational families, instead situating embodied distress as a result of broader political economies of migration and examining how intergenerational care relations foster family unity despite distance and physical separation (Yarris 2015). My perspective on young people living in families rendered vulnerable to forced separation through deportation is therefore informed both by the trauma invoked by state immigration policies but also how family members draw on intergenerational care and solidarity as cultural resources for survival.

Sanctuary Politics in Oregon

Against this backdrop of increasing public awareness of and protest against family separation as a centerpiece of federal immigration policy, migrant rights' activists have increasingly targeted state and local policies as possibilities for immigrant protection and inclusion. This is the case in Oregon, where the meanings and boundaries of the state's 1987 sanctuary law have re-emerged as important sites for legal and political organizing. The first state in the United States to pass "sanctuary" legislation, Oregon passed ORS 181A.820 in 1987 with broad bipartisan support in the state legislature and from both the business and immigrant rights communities (Oregon Laws 2022). The law prohibited the use of state or local resources or law enforcement personnel in pursuit of federal immigration enforcement activities (Wilson 2018). In an ongoing research endeavor, I am examining the past and present of Oregon's sanctuary policies from a social movement perspective, engaging as a participant-observer in a number of local and statewide organizations and campaigns that seek to both defend the law and to adapt it to current political realities.

Sanctuary has been productively critiqued by a number of US and UK scholars on a number of grounds. One set of critiques focuses on the ways "sanctuary" may offer a false sense of security to migrants and refugees in local polities while failing to address broader state exclusionary policies, and also perhaps masking deeper historical racialized power inequalities (Bagelman 2013). In a more positive rendering, Linda Rabben (2016) has described how sanctuary movements in the United States since the early 2000s have mobilized local volunteers to find creative ways of supporting immigrant integration, migrants' rights, and refugee resettlement. Germane to the present discussion, these modes of sanctuary activism include local efforts to "disentangle" state and local law enforcement from federal immigration enforcement activities (Rabben 2011: 214). While a broader examination and critique of contemporary sanctuary efforts is beyond the scope of the present chapter, here I engage with sanctuary as a social movement of local residents, activists, and allies advocating for greater protections for (im)migrant families and communities.

In Oregon, the state sanctuary law was challenged in the 2018 general elections by a ballot measure (Measure 105) that would have overturned the state's 1987 law. With backing from national anti-immigration organizations, Measure 105 was placed on the ballot by an ad hoc group calling itself Oregonians for Immigration Reform. Proponents, drawing on discourse circulating nationally on far-right and white nationalist websites, argued that the sanctuary statute acted as a "magnet," drawing undocumented immigrants from other states to Oregon where they supposedly took advantage of the state's friendly political climate to utilize social services and contribute to increased crime rates (Southern Poverty Law Center 2019). Opponents of Measure 105 came together in defense of the 1987 sanctuary statute under the umbrella "One Oregon," and included CAUSA, Oregon's statewide immigrant-rights organization, along with education, labor, and student organizations. One Oregon rolled out a grassroots organizing strategy, which included phone-banking and door-knocking, focusing their opposition to Measure 105 largely on the grounds that if the measure were to pass (and the sanctuary law were to be overturned), the state would see much higher rates of racial profiling by local law enforcement. After months of organizing, Measure 105 was resoundingly defeated, with 67 percent of Oregonians voting against (i.e., in favor of upholding the state's 1987 law). The margins against Measure 105 were highest in the state's largest cities: Portland, Salem, and Eugene. In Lane County, where Eugene is located and the ethnographic site of this chapter, the margin of opposition to Measure 105 was 68 percent to 32 percent ("Oregon Measure 105" 2018). The election results indicated that a majority of Oregonians supported the 1987 law and opposed the use of state and local law enforcement resources to engage in immigration enforcement activities.

This is important background for understanding the public testimony I analyze below, because the Lane County public hearing was called in response to residents' accusations that the county sheriff was collaborating with federal immigration enforcement efforts in violation of the state's sanctuary provisions. In early 2019, it had come to the attention of community organizations and immigrant rights activists that the Lane County sheriff was routinely allowing ICE (Immigration and Customs Enforcement) agents access to the county courthouse and jail. This collaboration purportedly included notifying ICE before people would be released from jail. Sounding the alarm, community leaders came together in early winter 2019 to write an open letter opposing this practice, which was published in the local newspaper, the *Eugene Register-Guard*.[1] The letter's fourteen signatories included directors of local non-profit social service organizations serving the Latinx community, staff at the ACLU of Oregon, and the Executive Director of CAUSA, among other community leaders. The letter alleged that sheriff's deputies were routinely contacting ICE and notifying these federal agents of the pending release of individuals about whom ICE might have "an interest," meaning, the individual might be eligible for deportation. A further aggravation to local activists, sheriff's deputies were allowing ICE agents special access to the county jail through a back entrance for the purposes of facilitating immigration arrests. The letter explicitly stated that these practices were in violation of Oregon state's sanctuary statute and reminded the sheriff that the use of local law enforcement resources for federal immigration enforcement activities is a violation of state law.

Mobilizing to Testify

After the letter to the sheriff was published, local activists called for a mass community mobilization to attend a Lane County Board of Commissioners meeting in order to register public testimony in opposition to the sheriff's collaboration with ICE. So it was that hundreds of community members gathered on a cold and cloudy midweek afternoon in February 2019 at the county offices building. A diverse cross-section of community members of various ages and ethnicities crowded into long rows of chairs that had been placed in a semi-circle facing the tall wooden bureau of benches behind which sat the five, all white and middle-aged, county commissioners. The tenor of the hearing, as articulated by activists ahead of time, was not to be overly confrontational, but rather to respectfully register the ways in which the sheriff's practices were: (a) directly and negatively impacting immigrant communities and (b) a violation of the state's sanctuary law. While hundreds of community members showed up to the hastily called public hearing, activists had sent out messages via social media prior to the meeting, indicating that only those "directly impacted community members" should sign up to testify, to allow space for the voices of those most-impacted by the threats of deportation and family separation. As a community member, ally, and engaged participant-observer, I did not put my name on the speaker's list. Instead, I sat and listened during the hearing as a range of community members shared their public testimony, including local residents who spoke in support of their neighbors, immigration attorneys, organizers with the statewide immigrant rights organization, CAUSA, directors of nonprofit, Latinx-serving, organizations, and students from both the local community college and the public university where I work.

As Briggs (1997: 521) signals, institutions structure testimony via constraints on audience, narrative structure, and content. In this county hearing, speakers were allowed three minutes each to testify, testimony would be given in the order that speakers signed up, and speakers gave their testimony while standing at the front of the hearing room behind a podium, facing the Commissioners, their backs to the public chamber. One remarkable element of this narrative structure is that public speakers have three minutes to speak, uninterrupted, and the commissioners are forced to assume the role of listener (Stephen 2017), sitting through powerful emotional testimony that they cannot turn away from or silence but must literally hear, head-on. Most speakers read from written remarks they have prepared ahead of time, a few spoke more informally. All speakers used the microphone and all oral testimony that day, which lasted for nearly two hours, was archived into the public record. As this was a public hearing, I was able to audio-record speakers using my IPhone's Voice Memo application. I later transcribed speakers' testimony verbatim, using my field notes and memory to recall non-verbal aspects of speech, emotional texture and tone, and notable aspects of audience response. My analysis of the testimony below focuses on the primary theme of interest to this chapter, namely, the ways in which several speakers articulated a particular subject position as "victim of family separation" as the grounds upon which to instantiate their political subjectivity.

Surviving Family Separation: Asserting a Right to Belong

One of the first speakers to give testimony at the Board of Commissioners meeting was Narisa,* director of a local non-profit organization serving the Latinx community (*all names are pseudonyms, despite this being public testimony, in order to protect speakers' identities). Narisa started by giving an overview of the state's sanctuary law and the protections it is supposed to give local communities from the types of practices the County Sherriff was engaging in. She referenced ORS 181.A20, the sanctuary law, and the "disentanglement" requirement that local law enforcement resources cannot be used for federal immigration enforcement purposes. Narisa referenced one particularly egregious case of information-sharing, in which the county sheriff had notified ICE when a local resident appeared for court-mandated alcohol treatment, leading to his detention. Narisa emphasized not only the injustice of these practices, but also the broader fear and insecurity that spread in the community as a result. She concluded,

> So if people don't feel safe there [at the courthouse], that fear spreads throughout the town and the county. So for me, running a non-profit, I want to see that our county is creating safe spaces, welcoming spaces, and this speaks volumes, if we allow this kind of interaction between the county, the sheriff's department, and Immigration [ICE].

Narisa spoke on behalf of the community, not as a victim of family separation or someone directly impacted by anti-immigrant policies, but as an advocate for the immigrant community. Narisa called for greater trust between residents and local law enforcement, but placed the responsibility for building that relationship squarely at the feet of the County Board of Commissioners, who oversee the sheriff's office and county law enforcement funding and activities. Her testimony was attention-grabbing, as she is a highly respected community leader, and she spoke in a forthright but convincing manner. Narisa made it clear to the commissioners that community organizations and allies were watching the sheriff's practices closely and calling on the Board to hold him accountable.

Another speaker to step to the podium at the County Commissioners' meeting was Jessica. Identifying herself as a social worker at a community non-profit organization, Jessica made the following, brief, statement:

> I am a survivor of family separation in the early [19]80s. I am a survivor of family separation in the mid-[19]90s. In 2019, I am still a survivor of family separation. To me, family means no one gets left behind or forgotten. I am here, I care, and I will take action for my family and my community. Growing up, I thought that the police was here to serve and protect, and now, how do I tell my children that the police are separating our families? Thank you.

As the first speaker of the morning, although Jessica's testimony was short (she left the podium before her three minutes were expired), it visibly moved the audience, who quieted down and listened, casting their eyes to the podium at the front of the room. The commissioners stared at Jessica, eyes unblinking, as if they had not anticipated this level of clarity in the testimony to be given that day. Of particular power in Jessica's narrative is that she identified herself as a "survivor of family separation" in the 1980s and 1990s. This was a powerful rhetorical reminder of the fact that family separation policies are not new, and that the state has been enacting violence on families through deportation and forced removals of parents for decades. Additionally, Jessica renders herself as a "survivor" of state violence, positioning her contemporary community activism as an outgrowth of her previous, firsthand, experience of family separation. Finally, Jessica's testimony highlights the ways family separation practices impact not just individuals subject to deportation and state removal but families, parents, and children, across generations. Having lived through family separation in the past, Jessica remarks on how it informs her role as a mother/parent in the present. Her testimony thus makes visible the ways the trauma of family separation is not only related to an event (initial detection, detention, or removal/deportation), but also to the ongoing, lasting consequences of separation.

Jessica's testimony evidences the fear and mistrust that spread within the community when word gets out that local law enforcement is collaborating with ICE. Jessica speaks to her diminished trust in local police, a hesitancy she is passing on to her children. But hers is not merely a trauma narrative, for Jessica inverts her positionality as a victim of family separation and claims survivorship as grounds for her current political subjectivity, as a mother, community member, professional, and an advocate for the immigrant community. In her very brief testimony, Jessica powerfully asserts her right to belong in this community and to assert herself as a politically active subject.

Toward the end of the public comment period, after more than an hour of testimony, two university students, Mayra and Antonio, came up to speak. Both of them powerfully employed the narrative positionality of "victim of family separation" to assert their political agency and their right to community belonging. Approaching the podium after a commissioner had incorrectly pronounced her name in calling her forward, Mayra's tone was somewhat curt and antagonistic, even as she followed the rules of respect and decorum structuring the public hearing, speaking within her allotted time and reading her prepared testimony. Here is an extract of her impassioned testimony:

> I am also a proud daughter of immigrants and as a daughter of immigrant parents, I have been taught since a young age to *ayudar a la comunidad y a los menos afortunados*, to help my community and those less fortunate. This has resonated with me still to this day as I have seen my immigrant community become the targets of anti-immigrant movements in the state of Oregon and across the nation. Releasing fear in our communities as a mechanism of control and making our local police do the job of federal law enforcement when they need to be making sure that they are keeping our communities safe. This practice violates even more of the little trust that exists between law enforcement and the public. We deserve answers and a commitment to the public by the Lane County sheriff that ends [the practice of] assisting ICE. And in the case that the Lane County sheriff's office does not stop violating the law, we will not stop fighting for the rights of our immigrant community. As some of you all know, and the sheriffs know, we are not quiet, and we will not be silent about this because local police working with ICE is against what we voted on and what represents us. Thank you.

Mayra's testimony was powerfully and emotionally delivered. While Mayra doesn't locate herself as a victim or survivor of family separation policies, she situates her political subjectivity squarely within her positionality as a "daughter of immigrant parents." Identifying collectively with her family and her "immigrant community," Mayra speaks to her commitment to advocate on behalf of those "menos afortunados," who include precariously statused immigrants. Mayra is forceful and angry when she describes the sheriff's practices of collaboration with ICE, and, like Narisa and Jessica before her, her testimony makes the consequences of these practices—namely, increased fear and decreased trust in the community—vividly clear to the commissioners. As Mayra spoke, I wondered whether her angry and agitated tone and her blue-colored hair might distance her from the commissioners, lessening the impact of her testimony. While I cannot be certain about how her words were received by the Board, the audience silently but powerfully registered their support as she stepped away from the podium, vigorously snapping their fingers in the air. Furthermore, Mayra's speech refuses a position of marginality, as she articulates her right to belong and to speak precisely because she is a child of immigrants. Her testimony also registers her political power as a member of the immigrant student movement, who, Mayra says, "will not be silent . . . [and] will not stop fighting."

After Mayra spoke, the next person to approach the podium was Antonio, who self-identified as an Oregon native, a third-year university student, and "a concerned Latinx and a citizen, and as the survivor of the effects of an ICE detention." Antonio also situated himself as a survivor of the harmful effects of immigration policies such as family separation as a means of asserting his legitimacy as a political subject with a particular right and claim to weigh in on local immigration policies. Antonio describes the breach of trust that has occurred between local law enforcement and Latinx communities, stating:

> As a Latinx, I do not feel comfortable enough to call police when there is an emergency. Prior to recent events highlighted in the media about police brutalities, I would have put my trust onto the police force, but they have lost my trust multiple times. Nobody should have to be afraid to call the police. What our sheriff has done highlights and has led to mistrust.

This was emotionally powerful testimony, using personal mistrust about the police to call out the problems of broader community breaches in safety and policing. Antonio's testimony illustrates how national high-profile cases of police brutality have created rifts in local communities, leading to less trust and less communication with local law enforcement.

Antonio referenced the support of Lane County voters for sanctuary policies. Emphasizing the resounding defeat of Measure 105, Antonio asserted: "The people have spoken and the sheriff, as a public servant, has an obligation to see that the law is respected." Antonio's political claim here is powerful because he references public support for sanctuary demonstrated in a statewide election as the backdrop in which the local county sheriff is operating, and violating, this public trust. Antonio thus moves from a position of mistrust of law enforcement to a strong political claim that the sheriff, as a public official, has an obligation to serve the community, by not using local law enforcement resources to collaborate with ICE.

After making these claims, the final minute of Antonio's testimony turned back to his self-presentation as a "survivor of family separation." Given the emotional weight and political power of his public testimony, I present his words verbatim here:

> I am also here as a survivor of the effects of family separation and an ICE detention. A decade ago, I came home from school to find that my mom had been detained. My little sister and I have not been able to completely recover from the effects of this incident. It is painful to come home and find that the one person you trust with your life is missing. The one person who was supposed to be there to love, nurture, and protect you from all harm can't be there and has not been able to be there for us because of ICE. ICE has brought an ICEstorm into my heart and that ICEstorm continues to wreak havoc within me as I stand here expressing my concerns. An ICEstorm that is fueled by the uncertainty of what the next day will entail. Will the call I receive from my parents bring up another detention? Does my parents' not answering their phone mean that they've been detained? If I miss my parents' call, I hope that they're OK, anytime they call me, I feel afraid that that maybe they're calling me because they've been detained or because they're in jail. When my mom was detained, we didn't even get to go to say "hi" to her, or say "bye" to her or anything. And we didn't see her after that for a whole year. [tearful pause] Thank you.

As Antonio stepped away from the podium, most in the packed hearing room again raised their fingers in silent snaps and waves, indicating their solidarity and support of what he had just said. In his short testimony in front of a packed public hearing room in a drab county office building, Antonio's narrative moved the audience emotionally and metaphorically toward understanding the trauma of family separation in a visceral way, as violence perpetrated against individuals, families, and communities, over time and across generations. His testimony, particularly the image of the "ICEstorm" and of the child uncertain whether their parent would be home to receive their phone call or would be deported by the state, also evoked images circulating in the media over the prior year of children held in detention at the border, crying, confused, and unclear about where their parents would be taken or what their future would hold. For a brief three minutes, Antonio's testimony transported the audience toward empathy with "victims of family separation" and families impacted by "ICEstorms" in a way that moved beyond news headlines and brought the impacts of these policies home, to the local community, through the story of one particular family. Vividly using the description of an "ICEstorm" to describe his family's experience of forced separation due to immigration enforcement policies, Antonio's testimony tied narrative directly to violence, forcing the audience into a reckoning with the effects of ICE practices on the lives of families. Antonio left no doubt as to the traumatic consequences of family separation for himself, his family, his relationship with his mother, and his sense of security. The image of not knowing whether his mother would be home when he called was a powerful reminder of the persistent uncertainty that immigrant families face in an era of political hostility, ICE raids, and mass detention and deportation.

Of course, there is a tension in this narrative display, particularly if it reinforces the victimhood of immigrant children rather than allowing for their agency as political subjects. This tension is what Lisa Malkki writes of in her astute critique of humanitarian work with children, which, as she shows, reduces children to victims in need of protection by the humanitarian regime, a move that elides young people's agency but also can pit children against their parents or blame parents for failing to protect children. While the US government's family separation policies have been placed under much scrutiny and protest, popular discourse still tends to focus on migrants and asylum seekers as victims of state violence, emphasizing harms done to "innocent children or families" (Malkki 2010). Miriam Ticktin has productively theorized the role of innocence within contemporary neoliberal humanitarian formations, arguing that, as innocence has "worked to produce the idea of a deserving humanity," it has simultaneously excluded the possibility of a "thinking, engaged, active, or informed subject" (Ticktin 2017: 579). With these critiques of victimhood and innocence in mind, here I seek to draw attention the ways a popular framing of family separation policies may unwittingly reinforce victimhood and deny migrants' full political personhood. In contrast, Antonio's testimony demonstrates how activists use public narrative to move beyond suffering and victimhood toward solidarity and recognition.

Antonio, Mayra, and other children of immigrant parents claim the space of public testimony not as victims but as young people demanding to be heard and recognized as political subjects. As Antonio's three minutes of testimony was running short, he concluded with the words "We didn't see her after that for a whole year," a vivid reminder of the duration of impacts following the event of an ICE raid (see also Lopez 2019). Again, Antonio's testimony was a narrative reminder of the embodied impacts of family separation, on parents and children, over time, and across generations. The "ICEstorm" that forced separation into Antonio's family disavows the "luxury" of talking about violence in a way that separates "narratives of violence apart from their referents" (Briggs 2007: 322). In Antonio's testimony, violence is made visible, through his words, through his person, and through his political presence. Antonio's testimony turned his personal past experience of surviving family separation (ICE's detention and deportation of his mother) into the grounds for his political subjectivity in the present. He narratively collapses the distance between violence and agency, claiming his identity as the survivor of an "ICEstorm" as the grounds upon which he asserts his right to speak out as a political subject. This testimony thus instantiates the intergenerational trauma of family separation, but also demonstrates how trauma can be transformed narratively into the grounds for an assertive and powerful political subjectivity.

Testimony and the Possibilities of Political Belonging

My primary purpose of participating in the public testimony on that day in February 2018 was as a concerned community member, participant active in several immigrant rights' groups in the community, and ally to folks impacted by the sheriff's collaboration with ICE. While I sat in the hearing, however, I felt the moral weight of bearing witness to the power of these public testimonies. I was moved to do more with these stories, because the narrative shift they contained—from victim to political subject—seemed to contain important narrative and political potential. To put it simply, this testimony demanded to be heard, and sharing it as an example of how local communities are mobilizing and using sanctuary policies to forge spaces of inclusion during exclusionary and hostile times is to me not just important to anthropological theorizing of migrant health and well-being, but also to broader public notions of community, belonging, and citizenship. Like Briggs describes his response to Ms. Gómez's testimony, as an anthropologist and observer, "she swept away the narrative ground on which I intended to stand—as interpreter, advocate, perhaps hero" (Briggs 2007: 316). As an engaged anthropologist and a community member, I expected to participate in the public hearing as an ally, my presence a sign of solidarity with local immigrant communities. I did not expect, however, to find myself so profoundly moved by the narrative testimonies that day, which "swept away" the narrative grounds upon which I had come to stand in relation to my understandings of family separation policies and their impacts on membership in political communities.

My intention in this chapter has been to reflect upon the power of this public testimony, on the narrative and political potential of testimony to resignify violence and victimhood and to assert the grounds for political membership and belonging. The testimony presented here challenges anticipated narratives of victimhood on multiple levels. First, the public context of this speech matters, as these young activists are giving voice to migrant suffering for the purpose of registering a political complaint and of making space for their political subjectivity. In the public hearing room in which their testimony was given, their narratives claimed space, not just on the docket of speakers for the county legislative session, but a space of belonging within a broader political community. As the crowd and the commissioners listened to their impassioned narratives, it was as if Mayra, Antonio, and the other speakers insisted on their rights to full membership in the community.

The creative narrative framing in this public testimony—"survivors of family separation"—makes the effects of state policies that forcibly separate families through detention and deportation vividly clear and impossible to deny. What otherwise might seem like abstract policies are narratively given embodied form, with testimony illustrating the traumatic impacts of state policies on individual bodies and subjectivities as well as on extended families. The latter point is key, as the narratives analyzed here insist on visibilizing the effects of violent state policies not just on individual subjects, but on family relationships, over generations and time.

Furthermore, in this narrative rendering, migrant victimhood becomes the grounds not just to seek protection but to demand rights as full political subjects, a political subjectivity that is demanded even as it not recognized by the state. In this way, these public testimonies employ a narrative pivot, away from victimhood and toward lived experience of state violence as grounds for political subjectivity. This narrative move is therefore both politically and analytically important for anthropologists of migration and health, who often find themselves in the troubling position of reaffirming migrant victimhood as the basis upon which deservingness to social services and political rights can be rendered. Here, my interest has been following how activists demand a space to belong on more universal grounds, not only through claims to suffering or victimhood. In my reading then, these narratives contain the potential for a radical reframing of political subjectivity—a mode of being authorized not on the basis of legal documentation but rather on the basis of lived experience, recognition, and a right to belong. Furthermore, these activists assert their right to belonging should not come at the cost of their parents, but rather be viewed as an intergenerational right—earned through their parents' sacrifice and presented as a collective, familial right to membership in the political community.[2]

Put another way, this chapter has traced how immigrant rights activists articulate their relationship to the state as both victims of violent policies that have separated families through immigrant policing and deportation but also as active members of local communities who demand their right to political belonging. I have examined how public testimony enables the visibility of migrant suffering but also asserts political agency and articulates novel forms of immigrant belonging. I have focused on how activists use public testimony against local law enforcement collaboration with ICE as a space through which to re-narrativize their positionality as "survivors of family separation," in other words, as rights-bearing, legitimate political subjects with powerful claims to political recognition and belonging. Through this analysis, we see how migrant testimony contains the possibility of reframing abject positionalities into new forms of political subjectivities premised on the right to belong precisely because of lived experiences of state violence. As I witnessed the public hearing of the Board of Commissioners, in a packed county hearing room, for a few hours at least, the noise of the media, executive tweets about the criminality of migrants, and other forms of depersonalized violence receded into the background as speakers made visible the impacts of state policy on immigrant families and communities. But speakers also used their narrative testimony as an opportunity to move beyond victimhood, reframing themselves as political agents, and reclaiming their rights to political membership and belonging, even as their legal status remains precarious. Narrative testimony becomes grounds upon which to reimagine migrant subjectivity and political belonging in hostile times.

Acknowledgments

Much appreciation goes to CAUSA for their work on behalf of immigrant communities in Oregon. Thank you to my former students Samantha Sidline and Brenda Garcia-Millan for comments on earlier versions of this chapter and for assistance with manuscript preparation. I am honored and grateful that Nadia and Stéphanie included my work in this important volume.

Kristin Elizabeth Yarris is an associate professor of global studies at the University of Oregon, where she is on the faculty steering committee and is former Director of the Global Health Program. Her research and teaching focus on transnational migration, global health, and global mental health. At UO, Kristin is affiliated faculty with the

Department of Anthropology and the Department of Women's, Gender, and Sexuality Studies. She also serves on the steering committees for the Center for the Study of Women and Society and the UO Dreamers Working Group.

Notes

1. Letter from Community leaders to Sheriff Byron M. Trapp, 1 February 2019. Accessed 24 July 2019 from https://www.documentcloud.org/documents/5733276-Sheriff-Trapp-Open-Letter-ICE-Policies.html.
2. This collective framing aligns with the strategies of immigrant youth activists in the United States who have advocated for a Dream Act, offering a pathway to legal residency or naturalized citizenship, not just for themselves as the Dreamer generation, but for their parents and extended families. These activists have resisted pitting their individual deservingness against their parents' and insisted on their political agency against broader political forces that would position them as "victims" of their parents' decisions to come to the United States, for instance. For an excellent historical examination of the Dreamers movement in the United States, see Wides-Muñoz (2018).

References

Bagelman, Jennifer. 2013. "Sanctuary." *Alternatives: Global, Local, Political* 38(1): 49–62.

Blommaert, Jan. 2001. "Investigating Narrative Inequality: African Asylum Seekers Stories in Belgium." *Discourse & Society* 12(4): 413–49.

Briggs, Charles. 1997. "Notes on a "Confession": On the Construction of Gender, Sexuality, and Violence in an Infanticide Case." *Pragmatics* 7(4): 519–46.

———. 2007. "Mediating Infanticide: Theorizing Relations between Narrative and Violence." *Cultural Anthropology* 22(3): 315–56.

Caple James, Erica. 2004. "The Political Economy of 'Trauma' in Haiti in the Democratic Era of Insecurity." *Culture, Medicine and Psychiatry* 28(2): 127–49.

Carling, Jørgen, and Francis Collins. 2018. "Aspiration, Desire and Drivers of Migration." *Journal of Ethnic and Migration Studies* 44(6): 909–26.

Families Belong Together. 2019. "Families Belong Together." Retrieved 25 July 2019 from https://www.familiesbelongtogether.org/about/.

Fassin, Didier, and Estelle d'Halluin. 2005. "The Truth from the Body: Medical Certificates as Ultimate Evidence for Asylum Seekers." *American Anthropologist* 10(4): 597–608.

Habbach, Hajar, Kathryn Hampton, and Ranit Mishori. 2020. "'You Will Never See Your Child Again': The Persistent Psychological Effects of Family Separation." *Physicians for Human Rights*, 25 February 2020. Retrieved 9 January 2022 from https://phr.org/our-work/resources/you-will-never-see-your-child-again-the-persistent-psychological-effects-of-family-separation/.

Kline, Nolan. 2019. *Pathogenic Policing: Immigration Enforcement and Health in the U.S. South.* New Brunswick, NJ: Rutgers University Press.

Kvittingen, Anna, Marko Valenta, Hanan Tabbara, Dina Baslan, and Berit Berg. 2018. "The Conditions and Migratory Aspirations of Syrian and Iraqi Refugees in Jordan." *Journal of Refugee Studies* 32(1): 106–24.

Lopez, William D. 2019. *Separated: Family and Community in the Aftermath of an Immigration Raid.* Baltimore, MD: Johns Hopkins University Press.

Malkki, Lisa. 2010. "Children, Humanity, and the Infantilization of Peace." In *In the Name of Humanity: The Government of Threat and Care*, ed. Illana Feldman and Miriam Ticktin, 58–85. Durham, NC: Duke University Press.

Musalo, Karen. 2019. "Evolution of Refugee and Asylum Law in the United States." In *Refugees and Asylum Seekers: Interdisciplinary and Comparative Perspectives*, ed. S. Megan Berthold and Kathryn R. Libal, 17–43. Santa Barbara, CA: Praeger.

Oregon Laws. 2022. ORS 181A.820. Enforcement of federal immigration laws. Retrieved 20 January 2022 from: https://oregon.public.law/statutes/ors_181a.820.

Oregon Measure 105. 2018. "Oregon Measure 105: Repeal Sanctuary State Law Initative." Retrieved July 26 2019 from https://ballotpedia.org/Oregon_Measure_105,_Repeal_Sanctuary_State_Law_Initiative_(2018).

Rabben, Linda. 2016. *Sanctuary & Asylum: A Social and Political History*. Seattle: University of Washington Press.

———. 2011. *Give Refuge to the Stranger: The Past, Present, and Future of Sanctuary*. Walnut Creek, CA: Left Coast Press.

Southern Poverty Law Center. 2019. "Federation for American Immigration Reform." Retrieved 26 July 2019 from https://www.splcenter.org/fighting-hate/extremist-files/group/federation-american-immigration-reform.

Stephen, Lynn. 2017. "Bearing Witness: Testimony in Latin American Anthropology and Related Fields." *The Journal of Latin American and Caribbean Anthropology* 22(1): 85–109. https://doi.org/10.1111/jlca.12262.

Ticktin, Miriam. 2017. "A World without Innocence." *American Ethnologist* 44(4): 577–90. https://doi.org/10.1111/amet.12558.

US Citizenship and Immigration Services. 2015. "Individual Seeking Asylum: Questions and Answers: Credible Fear Screening." Last modified 15 July 2015. Retrieved 9 January 2022 from https://www.uscis.gov/humanitarian/refugees-and-asylum/asylum/questions-and-answers-credible-fear-screening.

US Department of Health and Human Services. 2019. "Separated Children Placed in Office of Refugee Resettlement Care." Reports. Retrieved 25 July 2019 from https://oig.hhs.gov/oei/reports/oei-BL-18–00511.pdf.

US Department of Justice. 2018. "Memorandum for Federal Prosecutors along the Southwest Border," media release. Retrieved 25 July 2019 from https://www.justice.gov/opa/press-release/file/1049751/download.

Watters, Charles. 2019. *Mental Health and Well-Being: Intercultural Perspectives*. London: Red Globe Press.

Wides-Muñoz, Laura. 2018. *The Making of a Dream: How a Group of Young Undocumented Immigrants Helped Change What It Means to Be American*. New York: Harper.

Wilson, Conrad. 2018. "Oregon Voters to Decide the Fate of State's Sanctuary Law." *Oregon Public Broadcasting*, 3 October 2018. Retrieved 26 July 2019 from https://www.opb.org/news/article/oregon-election-sanctuary-law-measure-105/.

Yarris, Kristin Elizabeth. 2014. "'Quiero Ir y No Quiero Ir' (I Want to Go and I Don't Want to Go): Nicaraguan Children's Ambivalent Experiences of Transnational Family Life." *The Journal of Latin American and Caribbean Anthropology* 19(2): 284–309.

———. 2015. "Grandmothers, Children, and Intergenerational Distress in Nicaraguan Transnational Families." In *Global Mental Health: Anthropological Perspectives*, ed. Brandon Kohrt and Emily Mendenhall, 117–34. Walnut Creek, CA: Left Coast Press.

———. 2017. *Care across Generations: Solidarity and Sacrifice in Transnational Families*. Stanford, CA: Stanford University Press.

Yarris, Kristin, and Heide Castañeda. 2015. "Special Issue Discourses of Displacement and Deservingness: Interrogating Distinctions between 'Economic' and 'Forced' Migration." *International Migration* 53(3): 64–69. https://doi.org/10.1111/imig.12170.

Yoon-Hendricks, Alexandria, and Zoe Greenberg. 2018. "Protests across U.S. Call for End to Migrant Family Separations." *New York Times*, 30 June. Retrieved 5 June 2019 from https://www.nytimes.com/2018/06/30/us/politics/trump-protests-family-separation.html.

Zayas, Luis H. 2015. *Forgotten Citizens: Deportation, Children, and the Making of American Exiles and Orphans*. Oxford: Oxford University Press.

Zayas, Luis H., Sergio Aguilar-Gaxiola, Hyunwoo Yoon, and Guillermina Natera Rey. 2015. "The Distress of Citizen-Children with Detained and Deported Parents." *Journal of Child and Family Studies* 24(11): 3213–23. https://doi.org/10.1007/s10826-015-0124-8.

Afterword

Heide Castañeda

The study of migration and health requires a recognition that mobility across borders affects every aspect of experience, with an almost complete realignment of daily life that has significant social, economic, and health consequences. As a public health priority, migration is increasingly an important focus for understanding and improving health and healthcare globally, requiring a consideration of large-scale forces including social inequality, political instability, economic insecurity, and climate change. These forces often produce patterned experiences for migrants in "host" countries, shaping their access to employment, housing and living conditions, food security, and legal status, with consequences for overall well-being (Castañeda et al. 2015). Migrants must thus traverse additional social, economic, political, historical, discursive, and ideological borders—beyond actual physical or geographical borders—in search of health.

Globally, people continue to be displaced by various combinations of violence, choice, and circumstance, challenging conventional ideas about "voluntary" migrants in search of opportunity, and "involuntary" migrants, who are forced to flee in search of physical security. Even those who move voluntarily generally do so because economically violent circumstances have obstructed life chances for them and their families. In other words, the causes of migration are complex and not easily characterized as either voluntary or involuntary (Yarris and Castañeda 2015). However, how we frame the migration has enormous social and legal ramifications. When migration is viewed as unusual or even pathological, assumptions are carried over into research as well as policy and practice. If migration is viewed as an expected, appropriate, and often necessary response to various forms of violence, it can result in the development of equitable policies to address disparities. This response requires a recognition of global patterns of inequality that foster migration that are ultimately based in social, political, and economic conditions.

In recent years, we have all grappled with the effects of a global pandemic that has highlighted the degree to which health across the world is interconnected, in addition to laying bare the cracks in healthcare systems and inequalities of contemporary forms of governance. As the COVID-19 pandemic unfolded, it became clear just how existing social and economic conditions as well as political decision-making based on nationalist, xenophobic principles rather than public health data can produce unprecedented death and destruction. The pandemic abruptly halted the movement of people and goods via border shutdowns and travel restrictions across the globe, some of which barred entry to anyone who is not a citizen or permanent resident of the country while others suspended access by people from certain regions. As we continue to account for the effects of COVID-19 and similar global health events, research must continue to focus on the various scales of human, economic, and disease mobility, as well as the international and internal borders that selectively open and close to different populations.

Yet even as attention focused on closing borders, migrant populations faced struggles in host countries in which they already live, offering lessons for the future as well. As a result of social distancing measures, many of the most vulnerable were left feeling condemned to total disappearance from the social life of their communities. Migrants frequently live in densely populated centers where they have higher rates of susceptibility to communicable disease. They tend to earn less, lack health insurance, and be unable to take paid sick leave (or work from a home office), all of which negatively impact outcomes. Further affecting convalescence, recovery, and spread of outbreaks, they may be unwilling to present to a hospital or engage with official testing sites and vaccination programs because of their migration status. Many, especially those who are undocumented or irregular, were excluded from government assistance programs, such as unemployment or cash stimulus payments; despite their contributions to economies worldwide, they missed out on aid meant to help communities weather the pandemic. Anti-immigrant rhetoric led to public harassment and discrimination, targeting certain groups such as Chinese communities. Furthermore, raids and deportations continued in many places, despite the shutdown of other governmental activities. In addition to diverting resources away from tackling the pandemic, these actions promoted additional fear and discouraged people from seeking out necessary medical evaluation or treatment.

On a global scale, many migrants found themselves stuck in transit sites during the pandemic, caught between home and their final destination. Others live in crowded refugee camps where—as in detention facilities worldwide—efforts at physical distancing to slow the spread of a respiratory virus are simply impossible. Finally, one of the lasting impacts of global events like pandemics is that they prompt new migration around the world, as people's livelihoods are affected and their communities are flattened by the social, demographic, and economic impacts of disease.

Migration and Health: Challenging the Borders of Belonging, Care, and Policy

This book has discussed the various borders—social, economic, political, historical, discursive, and ideological—of health and healthcare as they appear in the context of migration. As highlighted in the introduction, it is the selective permeability of borders that makes them particularly noteworthy and useful to think with to inform broader theoretical and practical concerns. Across the various chapters, scholars use ethnographic engagements to illustrate the impacts of policies on health in migrant communities. The first part of the book examined deservingness and constructions of legitimacy—the often less visible borders of belonging and exclusion—in a variety of national contexts. The second part explored how migrants' health status and needs may challenge the borders of biomedical care. Finally, the last section examined policy borders affecting migrant access to health and healthcare. In the remainder of this conclusion, I focus on some major themes that emerged across the various chapters of the book.

Structural Conditions Impacting Migrant Health

Several chapters engage extensively with structural conditions impacting migrant health, many of which are rooted in various forms of colonialism. These conditions include social determinants such as economic structures, policies, and institutions that produce upstream, macrolevel inequalities in employment, housing and living conditions, access to food and health services, as well as legal status.

Rebecca Walker and Elsa Oliveira illustrate, using the case of South Africa, how foreign-born nationals face high levels of xenophobic discrimination and thus indirect and direct structural violence, including difficulties accessing documentation and free public health care, challenges finding employment, life in poverty, and the hardships of parenting alone. Carolyn Sargent, Laurent Zelek, and Anne Festa highlight the intersection of economic and social precarity, polypathology, and existential vulnerability for migrants living in Paris, with implications for accessing health care. As they note, "Instability in residence, effect of treatment on capacity to work, decline in household revenue, difficulties obtaining childcare, may all converge with declining physical well-being to generate an unyielding border of constraint to care." Finally, in the chapter by Cristiana Giordano, we see how the nexus of migration and mental health warrants larger discussions of "culture," while accounting for the impacts of broader historical processes in Italian society. As she deftly reveals, interpretations and diagnostic categories of mental illness and cultural difference by health practitioners working with migrants in Italy are rooted in colonial and post-colonial conditions and constructions.

Deservingness

A major contribution of the various chapters is how the legitimacy or "deservingness" of migrant populations regarding health care is reckoned and experienced. As elaborated in the chapter by Sarah Willen and Jennifer Cook, conceptions of health-related deservingness are fundamentally expressed in a moral register, as vernacular expressions of value as opposed to rights. They offer a framework for grappling with identifying and responding to notions of deservingness by focusing on three core elements: the stakeholders involved, the contexts in which deservingness assessments take place, and the evaluative criteria employed. Particularly valuable is their examination of the third element, which focuses on who migrants are and what they do, or do not, deserve: evaluative criteria may include characteristics such as migration motive, legal status, moral character, vulnerability, and social proximity to members of the broader society.

As one example of this, in the chapter by Nolan Kline, we see deservingness play out sharply based on racially informed ideologies of what makes a particular type of migrant desirable. By examining two contrasting policy contexts—first, exclusions related to concerns about immigrants becoming a "public charge" or drain on public finances, and second, a visa policy that expedites authorized statuses to immigrants who invest large sums of money in the United States—this chapter highlights nativist notions of belonging that conflate race, citizenship, and health.

Listening to Migrants

Many of the chapters emphasize the importance of listening to migrants themselves. The case brought by Walker and Oliveira is especially powerful in illustrating how migrant women in South Africa, despite the weight of their everyday struggles, are key players in determining and influencing their own trajectories and the spaces they inhabit. In doing so, the authors seek to resist simple notions of victimhood and vulnerability, focusing instead on women's layered, complex lives. They describe the powerful psychological impact of "being seen"; that is, of having health care workers acknowledge, recognize, and treat them as deserving of care, a sort of antidote to the exclusions and "otherings" that happen in their daily lives.

Indeed, as Kristin Elizabeth Yarris points out in her chapter, in recent years there has been a move away from studies on suffering and victimhood and toward listening to migrants' hopes, aspirations, and desires. Here, she focuses on testimony as a particular performative narrative form, in which the goal is often to "capture a certain narrative formulation of migranthood," one that uses selective listening and is focused on hardship, suffering, and abuse. In this powerful piece, Yarris illustrates how migrants in the United States are able to resignify the narrative testimony of "victim of family separation" instead into a marker of political potentiality.

In sum, many of the authors remind us that scholars and policymakers must all learn to listen to migrants in their own words. As Willen and Cook ask: "What sort of social contracts do they perceive, envision, or hope for? . . . What barriers impede their ability to speak out and participate in these debates on their own behalf? . . . What are the health effects for migrants and their families of being made to feel unwelcome and undeserving of society's attention, investment, or care?"

Listening to Those Who Care

Many of the chapters also foreground those who care for migrants, highlighting their perspectives, experiences, and voices. Giordano, for instance, describes the complex and ambivalent perspectives of ethnopsychiatrists in Italy, as they grapple with their discipline's fraught history and its implications for themselves and for those they treat. The chapter by Sargent, Zelek, and Festa focuses on an association in Paris that offers an exemplary model of health care provision for low-income immigrants; in doing so, it works to deconstruct borders designed to restrict access to health care institutions and sources of social support. Additionally, Rania Kassab Sweis, in a chapter that shifts ethnographic focus away from recipients to the providers of aid in the Syrian Civil War, examines the various racial and cultural hierarchies that exist within global humanitarianism and foregrounds the professional lives and situated practices of global aid workers.

Reproducing Crisis Narratives?

Finally, the work in this book collectively warns against reproducing narratives of crisis—something which, to return to the start of the chapter, is already on the horizon as scholars grapple with the impacts of COVID-19 and narratives that distract from the failures of our healthcare systems and contemporary governance systems based on inequality. The pandemic highlighted not only the important role of mobility but also of these selectively permeable borders. As scholars and practitioners, we frequently identify migration as a variable of interest, but it is an artificial one at best, as humans have always migrated and the health implications of doing so are not uniformly negative. This focus on crisis also fosters ideas of victimhood, which many of the chapters in this volume push against in order to avoid essentializing people's experiences. While contemporary migration has reached an unprecedented scale, we must avoid the pitfalls of reproducing these narratives. Most importantly, as the work in this book illustrates, it is the selective permeability of borders, whether they be social, economic, political, historical, discursive, and/or ideological, that fosters such narratives of crisis and exceptionality.

The Study of Migration and Health: Contributions from Anthropology

Anthropology, and specifically medical anthropology, is the primary grounding discipline for the authors in this edited volume. But why is anthropology particularly well-suited to larger discussions of migration and health? What is the added value of the anthropological perspective for other disciplines, for policy, and for practice?

Medical anthropology is a field that routinely challenges borders: borders between patients and clinicians, between individuals and communities, between biological sciences and humanistic experiences. We are repeatedly reminded in this volume of the need to challenge borders in order to take seriously migrant and healthcare provider experiences. Indeed, the anthropological study of migrant health forces us to rethink commonly held ideas and critically unravel conventional ideas of the connection between these topics. Notably, there is a conceptual tendency in public discourse to naturalize the global regime of nation-states. This produces an analytical bias that privileges often violent regimes of citizenship as the site for social processes, to the neglect of other kinds of experiences. Put another way, in our current global system, there is no stable epistemic partition between "here" and "there," and migrants are not simply dislocated, "displaced," or "uprooted" persons who demonstrate some form of "spatial disobedience" (DeGenova 2016).

Anthropological approaches warn us against this pitfall of the presumed stability of "located-ness" of populations. Otherwise, analyses of migrant health are easily reduced to simplistic and groundless abstractions about geographically originating cultural differences. Despite its everyday application in clinical and public health settings, "culture" is a complex and ambiguous domain, at best. Rather than simply leaving the issue unproblematized, anthropologists reflect upon how exaggerating the importance of culture can obscure broader structural determinants of health and pathogenic role of social inequality.

Instead, the study of migrant health from an anthropological perspective highlights social inequality in the global system. Migration is increasingly a low-cost, flexible, and legally vulnerable source of reserve labor for wealthy nations. Yet while "host" countries obtain all benefits, migrants are faced with structures that perpetuate deportability, violence, exploitation, and disability, and frequently deny them access to resources, let alone the possibility to fully integrate in host societies. Thus, the availability of healthcare resources becomes a lens for understanding the state's response to migration and uniquely highlights the body as a site for the inscription of politics and social legitimacy. In order to understand these experiences, medical anthropologists seek to account for the large-scale social and political forces that impact migrants, including global inequality, political instability, economic insecurity, and climate change. Inequities in the well-being of migrants are heavily determined by factors such as exclusionary policies, discrimination and racism, employment in marginal and dangerous jobs, the high cost of health care, inadequate housing, and poor access to transportation and other resources. As this volume highlights, anthropological approaches using long-term ethnographic fieldwork, locally situated analyses, and attention to the understandings of our interlocutors have contributed to a richer understanding of the relationship between migration and health.

As the chapters in this book have pointed out, analyses of migrant health require a focus on the social origins of illness and the context that precedes them, and particularly how inequality, poverty, institutional constraints, and violence contribute to disparities. This is because being a migrant is not in itself a risk to health; it relies upon the preexistence of certain kinds of vulnerabilities, which requires a critical lens for understanding. And of course, the experiences of migrants must also be understood as intersectional, since health-related opportunities as well as injustices and inequalities are enacted on a multidimensional basis dependent on factors such as racialization, ethnicity, gender, age, country of origin, sexual orientation, social class, and religion.

Future Directions

Finally, what are some future directions for scholars and practitioners concerned with migration and health? Where do we go from here?

First, we must always be mindful about how we frame the origins and reasons for migration. Researchers, practitioners, and policymakers alike must be acutely attentive to discourse in debates on migration and trouble notions of "deservingness" as they emerge. This requires a recognition that the global patterns of inequality fostering migration are not based on cultural difference, but are instead rooted in social, political, and economic conditions produced and reproduced by legal frameworks and institutions.

While other axes of health inequality, such as gender and race, are increasingly well-studied, migration as a unique variable remains understudied. Migrants experience specific impacts on health due to restricted access to care, structural constraints related to inequality, poverty, and housing and working conditions, as well as the stress associated with precarious legal status. Specific topical areas remain understudied, such as undocumented migrants' access to expensive but lifesaving care (such as major surgeries or transplants); clinical ethics and practical decision making by healthcare workers and administrators; unauthorized im/migration and reproductive politics; dental /oral health; and broader public health risks generated by the denial of care to unauthorized im/migrants. Furthermore, border control and law enforcement activities continue to increase in host countries, and researchers must continue to examine the health effects of these forms of violence as well.

Finally, it is a crucial time to consider the study of migration and health in a post-pandemic world in order to inform research, practice, and advocacy priorities. Will global migration slow down or speed up? How and why? Scholars of migration and health are used to studying people on the move, along with the state responses to this movement. However, global migration patterns increasingly characterized by immobility, as more people become stranded in destination countries, zones of transit, and refugee camps. Thus, a theoretical and practical focus on the effects of forced immobility and its relationship to health has become a priority. Furthermore, discourses about protecting public health are poised to replace securitization narratives that emerged post-9/11 for governments seeking to strengthen their external borders and limit immigration. Will public health increasingly be used as a rationale not only to control border crossings but to further disenfranchise communities postmigration? What will be the impacts on migrant communities, especially as they interplay with intensified surveillance and exclusionary policies? These are some of the crucial considerations moving forward as we take stock of the central importance of human mobility, interconnections across borders, and the persistence of social and economic inequality around the globe.

Heide Castañeda is a Professor of Anthropology at the University of South Florida. Her research areas include critical border studies, political and legal anthropology, medical anthropology, migration, migrant health, citizenship, focusing on the U.S./Mexico border, Mexico, Germany, and Morocco. She is the author of *Borders of Belonging: Struggle and Solidarity in Mixed-Status Immigrant Families* (Stanford University Press, 2019) and co-editor of *Unequal Coverage: The Experience of Health Care Reform in the United States* (NYU Press, 2018). Her latest book, *Migration and Health: Critical Perspectives*, is forthcoming with Routledge. Dr. Castañeda has also published dozens of research articles on migration and health care access for immigrant populations. Her work has been funded by the National Science Foundation, National Institutes of Health, the Fulbright Program, the German Academic Exchange Service (DAAD), and the Wenner-Gren Foundation for Anthropological Research.

References

Castañeda, Heide, Seth M. Holmes, Daniel S. Madrigal, Maria-Elena DeTrinidad Young, Naomi Beyerle, and James Quesada. 2015. "Immigration as a Social Determinant of Health." *Annual Review of Public Health* 36: 75–392.

De Genova, Nicholas. 2016. "The 'Native's Point of View' in the Anthropology of Migration." *Anthropological Theory* 16(2–3): 227–40.

Yarris, Kristin, and Heide Castañeda. 2015. "Discourses of Displacement and Deservingness: Interrogating Distinctions between Economic and Forced Migration." *International Migration* 53(3): 64–69.

Index

www.ingramcontent.com/pod-product-compliance
Ingram Content Group UK Ltd.
Pitfield, Milton Keynes, MK11 3LW, UK
UKHW042103180825
461986UK00008B/502

9 781800 73501